Research in Filariasis and Schistosomiasis

RESEARCH IN
FILARIASIS AND SCHISTOSOMIASIS

Volume 2

edited by
Muneo YOKOGAWA

UNIVERSITY PARK PRESS
Baltimore · London · Tokyo

UNIVERSITY PARK PRESS
Baltimore · London · Tokyo

Library of Congress Cataloging in Publication Data

United States-Japan Cooperative Medical Science Program.
  Japanese Working Group on Parasitic Diseases.
  Recent advances in researches on filariasis and schistosomiasis in Japan.

  Vol. 2 (1972) edited by M. Yokogawa has title: Research in filariasis and schistosomiasis, and imprint: Baltimore University Park Press.
  Includes bibliographies.
  1. Filaria and filariasis. 2. Schistosomiasis—Japan. I. Sasa, Manabu, 1916–   ed. II. Yokogawa, Muneo, 1918–   ed. III. Title. IV. Title: Research in filariasis and schistosomiasis. [DNLM: 1. Filariasis —Prevention and control—Japan. 2. Research— Japan. 3. Schistosomiasis—Prevention and control— Japan. WC 20 R432 1972]
RC142.5.U46   616.9'652   77-118666
ISBN 0-8391-0032-9 (v. 1)

Printed in Japan.
Originally published by
University of Tokyo Press

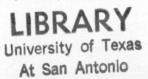

PREFACE

Parasitic diseases represent one of the areas on which the Joint Committee of the Japan-United States Cooperative Medical Science Program decided, in March 1965, to focus its attention. In accordance with this decision two panels were formed and the Japanese and United States delegations appointed as chairman for their respective panels Dr. Komiya and Dr. Jacobs, and subsequently assisted in the recruitment of panel members.

At the Honolulu Joint Conference in October 1965, the two panels on parasitic diseases agreed that they would focus on two major diseases of particular significance to the people of Asia, schistosomiasis and filariasis. It was decided that the following areas, which would be used as guide-lines, were of primary importance and merited intensive research.

Schistosomiasis
1. Pathogenesis including immunopathology
2. Pathology including biochemical and physiological studies of the parasites
3. Immunologic and serologic studies
4. Chemotherapy and pharmocological studies
5. Host-parasite relationship
6. Epidemiology and biological control

Filariasis
1. Animal transmission
2. Immunologic and serologic studies
3. Mosquito vectors
4. Chemotherapy
5. Epidemiology and biological control

These guidelines adopted by the two panels have been adhered to insofar as this is scientifically feasible, and as a result notable advances have been made in various areas. Those reports which were made during the four years after the organization of the Japanese working group were published in 1970 under the title "Recent

Advances in Researches on Filariasis and Schistosomiasis in Japan"
(edited by Dr. Manabu Sasa, former chairman of the Japanese
panel). However, due to a shortage of time allowed each worker
for preparation of the draft, some of the important works did not
meet the deadline and were ommitted.

This symposium was compiled as the second volume of "Recent
Advances in Researches on Filariasis and Schistosomiasis in Japan"
with the purpose of including the reports ommitted as well as the
reports prepared after the publication of the first volume.

Our grateful thanks are due to Dr. Toshio Kurokawa, chairman
of the Japanese Committee of the Japan-United States Cooperative
Medical Science Program, who gave his support and encouragement
to the activities of our working group, and to Dr. Ishimaru and his
associates in the Preventive Medicine Section, Ministry of Health
and Welfare, for assistance in organizing the panel and in the publication of this book. We are also indebted to Dr. Paul Weinstein
(chairman) and other members of the United States Panel on
Parasitic Diseases for their close collaboration in our research
activities.

This book was edited by panel members M. Yokogawa, M. Sasa,
K. Okabe, T. Ishizaki, and D. Katamine, with the cooperation of
the working group members.

The massive secretarial work of collecting and editing papers and
distributing proofs was handled by Dr. Hiroshi Tanaka and Dr.
Kazuo Yasuraoka.

We are greatly indebted to the staff members of the University of
Tokyo Press for their assistance in the publication of this book.

Muneo YOKOGAWA
Chairman, Japanese Panel

Tokyo Japan
May, 1972

Japanese Working Group on Parasitic Diseases, Japan-United States Cooperative Medical Science Program

Department of Parasitology, the Institute of Medical Science, University of Tokyo; Manabu SASA (Professor) and Hiroshi TANAKA (Associate Professor); Biology of mosquitoes and *Oncomelania* snails, immunology and experimental chemotherapy of filariasis and schistosomiasis, epidemiology of filariasis.

Department of Parasitology, National Institute of Health, Tokyo; Tatsushi ISHIZAKI (Chief), Kazuo YASURAOKA, and Toshio YANAGISAWA; Skin tests and other immunodiagnosis of schistosomiasis and filariasis, biology, biochemistry, and control of *Oncomelania* snails.

Department of Parasitology, School of Medicine, University of Chiba; Muneo YOKOGAWA (Professor), Motohito SANO (Associate Professor) and Somei KOJIMA (Lecturer); Epidemiology, immunology and chemotherapy of schistosomiasis.

Department of Endemic Diseases, Yamanashi Prefectural Institute for Public Health, Kofu, Haruhiko KUTSUMI (Chief); Epidemiology and control of schistosomiasis.

Department of Parasitology, School of Medicine, Gunma University; Toshisada SAWADA (Professor) and Koji ITO (Associate Professor); Immunology and antigen analysis in schistosomiasis and filariasis.

Department of Parasitology, Faculty of Medicine, Shinshu University, Matsumoto; Tomoo OSHIMA (Professor); Experimental studies on schistosomiasis.

Department of Parasitology, Faculty of Medicine, Yokohama City University; Shigeo HAYASHI (Professor) and Hisashi YAMAMOTO (Associate Professor); Epidemiology and immunology of filariasis.

Department of Parasitology, Juntendo University, School of Medicine, Tokyo; Hiroshi OYA (Professor); Biochemistry of schistosomes and *Oncomelania* snails.

Department of Parasitology, Okayama University, Medical School; Seiiti INATOMI (Professor); Electron-microscopic studies of schistosomes and filariae.

Department of Parasitology, Kurume University, School of Medicine; Koyo OKABE (Professor), Minoru AKUZAWA (Associate Professor); Epidemiology, control and immunology of schistosomiasis.

First Department of Pathology, Kurume University, School of Medicine; Toshiro NAKASHIMA (Professor) and Hiroshi TSUTSUMI (Associate Professor); Pathology of schistosomiasis.

First Department of Internal Medicine, Kurume University, School of Medicine; Makoto KURATA (Professor); Clinical studies on schistosomiasis.

Department of Parasitology, Institute for Tropical Medicine, Nagasaki University; Daisuke KATAMINE (Professor); Periodicity of microfilariae, skin tests in filariasis.

Department of Medical Zoology, Nagasaki University, School of Medicine; Yoshito WADA (Professor); Biology of mosquitoes in relation to transmission and epidemiology of filariasis.

Second Department of Internal Medicine, Faculty of Medicine, Kagoshima University; Hachiro SATO (Professor) and Yoshihito OTSUJI (Lecturer); Clinical and epidemiological studies on filariasis, electron-microscopic studies of filariae.

Department of Medical Zoology, Faculty of Medicine, Kagoshima University; Atsuo SATO (Professor) and Isao TADA (Associate Professor); Immunodiagnosis and epidemiology of filariasis.

Department of Tropical Disease Research, Research Institute of Tropical Medicine, Kagoshima University, Naze; Hideo FUKUSHIMA (Professor); Drug treatment and biochemical studies of filariasis.

Department of Medical Zoology, Faculty of Medicine, Hiroshima University; Moriyasu TSUJI (Professor); Immunology of schistosomiasis and filariasis.

Department of Parasitology, Faculty of Medicine, Kyushu University, Fukuoka; Kenjiro KAWASHIMA; Biological control of *Oncomelania* snails.

Department of Pathology, School of Medicine, University of Chiba; Tomio TADA; Immunology of schistosomiasis.

Department of Allergy, Institute of Medical Science, University of Tokyo; Tyoku MATUHASI (Professor); Immunology of filariasis.

Department of Parasitology, School of Medicine, Kyorin University; Toshihiko IIJIMA (Professor); Epidemiology of schistosomiasis.

Department of Medical Zoology, St. Marianna University School of Medicine; Tozo KANDA (Professor); Genetics of mosquitoes.

Department of Medical Zoology, School of Medicine, Nagoya City University; Shigefusa SATO (Professor); Immunology of schistosomiasis.

CONTENTS

CONTENTS

Research in Filariasis and Schistosomiasis

Epidemiology of Filariasis and Schistosomiasis in Asia and the Pacific: A Review*

M. SASA

Department of Parasitology, Institute of Medical Science,
University of Tokyo, Tokyo, Japan

INTRODUCTION

The Japan-United States Cooperative Medical Science Program, since it's establishment in 1965, has taken up the problems of parasitic diseases in Asia as a major subject of research, and panels have been organized in both countries to deal with this topic. It has been agreed that, for the time being, the activity of the panels be limited to only two parasitic diseases, filariasis and schistosomiasis.

In one activity under this project, I have been collecting information on the distribution and incidence of various parasitic diseases endemic in Asia. I think this information forms the most basic and important reference material for all aspects of research undertaken in this program. This paper is only a preliminary review based on results of surveys carried out by many workers in Asia, but I believe it to be sufficient for evaluating the importance of parasitic disease as a health hazard to people in Asia, and for emphasizing future research needs in this field of medicine.

As of 1970, Asia has a population of nearly 2 billion, or 56% of the total world's population (about 3.5 billion). It is divided into more than 20 countries of different races, religions and customs, in developing or underdeveloped stages of economic growth. The most highly populated areas are in the tropic zone where a variety of parasitic diseases are endemic. Furthermore, many of the parasitic diseases highly prevalent in Asia occur rarely, if at all, in civilized countries in the temperate zone, and are thus ignored by modern medicine.

---

* This study was conducted while a Fogarty Scholar-in-Residence, Fogarty International Center, NIH.

[3]

FILARIASIS

Filariasis is a great hazard to the health and welfare of people in Asia, and it is estimated to involve several hundred million people in its endemic areas which are scattered in almost all Asian countries. Furthermore, the status of filariasis in Asia and the Pacific is extremely complicated, but a great deal of information has been added recently to an understanding of its epidemiology. Two species of human filariae are known to be endemic in this region, *Wuchereria bancrofti* and *Brugia malayi*, the latter being indigenous only to southern and eastern Asia. Both species are further classified into "periodic" and "subperiodic" forms, which differ from each other in the periodicity of microfilariae, geographic distribution, and species of vector mosquitoes. Some forms are further divided into types or "sub-forms" associated with different epidemiological features and vector species, such as those seen in nocturnally periodic *W. bancrofti* and *B. malayi*. The "Timor-filaria" recently reported from Timor Island is possibly a third species (see Table 1).

Table 1.   Classification of Human Filariasis in the Asiatic-Pacific Region

Species of filaria	Periodicity type	Principal vector	Type of endemic area	Geographic distribution
Wuchereria bancrofti	Nocturnally periodic	*Culex pipiens* s. l.	urban	Japan, Okinawa, China, Indochina, Burma, India, Ceylon, E. Pakistan Maldive, Indonesia
		Aedes (Finlaya) poecilus	Abaca plantation	Philippines
		Anopheles spp.	rural	Philippines, Malaysia, Indonesia, New Guinea
	Nocturnally subperiodic	*Aedes (Finlaya) niveus*	rural	Thailand
	Diurnally subperiodic	*Aedes (Stegomyia)* spp.	urban and rural	South Pacific Islands
Brugia malayi	Nocturnally periodic	*Mansonia (Mansonioides)* spp.	rural	Indonesia, Malaysia, South Thailand, India, Ceylon, E. Pakistan
		Aedes (Finlaya) togoi	coastal	Japan (Hachijo-Koshima), Korea (Chejudo Is.), Continental China
	Nocturnally subperiodic	*Mansonia (Mansonioides)* spp.	jungle	Malaysia, Indonesia, Philippines
"Timor filaria"	Nocturnally periodic			Timor

Distribution of various types of filariasis

1. *Wuchereria bancrofti*, nocturnally periodic, transmitted by *Culex pipiens* s.l.

This is the most common and widely distributed form of filariasis in the world, and is known to be endemic in almost all Asian countries, including Japan, Ryukyu, Korea, continental China, Taiwan (mainly the Pescadores), the Philippines, Indonesian islands, West Malaysia, Vietnam, Laos, Burma, East Pakistan, India, Nepal, Ceylon, and Maldive. This type of filariasis is often called the urban form in contrast to the rural which is transmitted by jungle or swamp mosquitoes.

The principal vector of this form of filariasis is broadly *Culex pipiens* which includes various subspecies such as *fatigans* (=*quinquefasciatus*), *pallens* and *molestus*. The status of these forms in relation to geographic distribution, taxonomy, ecology and genetics was studied by Sasa *et al.* (1963–67). Although they differ from each other in some morphological and physiological characteristics, mosquitoes of this complex are all highly adapted for the development of *W. bancrofti* larvae and are similar in their biting and breeding habits, with the exception of the autogenous form of *molestus*. Their larvae breed mainly in sewage waters around houses, and are therefore widely spread in areas where the population density is especially high, such as the urban areas of developing countries.

The *fatigans*-borne bancroftian filariasis is highly prevalent in some South Asian countries. In India, for example, the population of endemic areas is estimated to be nearly 200 million, while that of continental China is considered to be almost the same size. The trends of rising incidence rates and widening range of endemic areas are especially marked in countries such as India, Burma, Ceylon and East Pakistan.

It should be noted also that the distribution and incidence of this form of filariasis are not necessarily related to the population density of the vector mosquitoes. This particular form of filariasis is almost absent from Thailand, Philippines, Malaysia and Taiwan, though the population density of *Culex pipiens fatigans* is very high in cities like Bangkok and Manila. On the other hand, it was surprising to see in Ceylon that the transmission of the disease had been efficiently maintained in environments with very few vector mosquitoes.

2. *Wuchereria bancrofti*, nocturnally periodic, transmitted by anopheline mosquitoes

In contrast to the mainly urban distribution of the *fatigans*-borne filariasis, rural forms of the nocturnally periodic bancroftian filariasis have also been reported from several South Asian countries. They are mainly transmitted by local anopheline mosquitoes that breed in swamps and streams. For example, filariasis widely distributed among people living in mountainous regions of West Malaysia was reported to be transmitted by *Anopheles maculatus, An. letifer* and *An. whartoni*, while *C. p. fatigans* was not suitable for the development of the parasite (Wharton, 1960; Ramachandran *et al.*, 1964). Bancroftian filariasis found in the mountain or jungle areas of Luzon and Palawan in the Philippines was shown to be transmitted by *An. minimum flavirostris* (Rozeboom and Cabrera, 1964, 1965). Such an anopheline-borne filariasis is also known to be endemic among natives of New Guinea, where *An. punctulatus* and other local species have been demonstrated to be the principal vectors.

3. *Wuchereria bancrofti*, nocturnally periodic, transmitted by *Aedes (Finlaya)* mosquitoes

Some species of the subgenus *Finlaya* of the genus *Aedes* have been known to act as excellent intermediate hosts of various forms of *W. bancrofti* and *B. malayi*, as was shown experimentally for *Aedes (Finlaya) togi*. A remarkable example of the occurrence of this type of filariasis is seen in the Philippine Islands, where the disease is mainly prevalent among people of the Abaca growing areas. There, the parasite is transmitted mainly by *Aedes (Finlaya) poecilus*, which has a peculiar habit of breeding in leaf axils of plants, such as Abaca and Banana.

4. *Wuchereria bancrofti*, nocturnally subperiodic

Bancroftian filariasis reported recently by Harinasuta *et al.* (1970, c) from a jungle zone of Thailand near the Burma border is apparently nocturnally subperiodic, and its principal vector is considered to be *Aedes (Finlaya) niveus*, a mosquito that breeds mainly in tree holes.

5. *Wuchereria bancrofti*, diurnally subperiodic, of the South Pacific islands

This has long been known to be different from the other forms in that the microfilariae are either nonperiodic, or diurnally subperiodic. It is also distinguished by the status of its principal vectors which belong to the day-biting species of the subgenus *Stegomyia* of the genus *Aedes*. A great deal of information has been accumulated by American and European workers, including Professor J. F. Kessel *et al.* (1957,

1960, 1962, 1966), in reference to the epidemiology and control of this form of filariasis.

The geographic distribution of this particular form of filariasis seems to be confined to a number of small islands located east of 170°, to about 120° east longtitude, and between 5°N and 25°S latitude. Microfilarial rates of over 20% or 30% have been reported from Fiji, Western and American Samoa, Cook, and Tahiti. Filariasis endemic in areas west of 170°E or in the Melanesian islands is, so far as we know, the nocturnally periodic type transmitted by the local anophelines.

Brugia malayi

In contrast to the worldwide distribution of the *Wuchereria bancrofti* infection, filariasis due to *Brugia malayi* is known only from South and East Asia. This parasite is known to have two forms, the nocturnally periodic and the nocturnally subperiodic; the former is further classified into two types according to the difference in the species of the principal vectors. Infection with the periodic form is apparently confined to human beings, while a number of animal reservoirs are known for the subperiodic form.

1. *Brugia malayi,* nocturnally periodic, transmitted mainly by *Mansonia (Mansonioides)* mosquitoes

This is apparently the most common type of Malayan filariasis found in tropical Asia, and has been reported from Indonesia (Sumatra, Java, Kalimantan, Celebes, Ceram), West and East Malaysia, southern Thailand, North Vietnam, southern China, India and Ceylon. The disease does not seem to have spread beyond the desert of West Pakistan, nor eastward beyond the strait separating Ceram Island and New Guinea. In most of these endemic areas, the swamp-breeding mosquitoes of the subgenus *Mansonioides* of the genus *Mansonia* act as the principal vectors. Their larvae have a peculiar habit of attaching to water plants with their siphon. The disease is therefore prevalent mostly among inhabitants of low and swampy areas. In some areas, local anopheline species have been confirmed as accessory vectors.

In general, the clinical symptoms seen in the acute stage, such as fever attacks and lymphangitis, are more severe in Malayan filariasis than in bancroftian. This type is associated with high elephantiasis rates, but does not cause genito-urinary signs, such as hydrocele and chyluria. The Malayan filariasis is especially prevalent among people

in some regions of India (especially the State of Kerala), southern
Thailand, and West Malaysia. In Ceylon, the disease was found to
be endemic in a number of areas when surveys were carried out during 1938–1948, but had almost disappeared from that country by
about 1955. It is assumed that the wide application of DDT residual
spraying in houses of the endemic areas carried out under the malaria
control project might have been effective also in the interruption of
transmission of Malayan filariasis.

2. *Brugia malayi*, nocturnally periodic, transmitted by *Aedes togoi*.

This type of Malayan filariasis was first found in Japan during a
survey carried out in 1950 by Hayashi, Sasa and others (1951, 1952)
on the small island of Hachijo-Koshima. The principal vector, *Aedes
(Finlaya) togoi*, breeds mainly in rock pools on the beach head, and is
therefore a disease attacking people living in the coastal regions. It
was later confirmed that the disease prevalent among inhabitants of
Chejudo Island of Korea and the coastal zones of continental China
is the same epidemiological type. *Aedes togoi* is a mosquito easily bred
in the laboratory, and has been found to be specially adapted for the
development of various filarial species, including *Wuchereria bancrofti*,
both periodic and subperiodic forms of *Brugia malayi* and other
Brugia species, and also *Dirofilaria immitis*. Thus it is now widely used
in experimental filaria studies. The larvae of *Aedes togoi* is characterized physiologically by its capacity for growing in water of high salt
content, such as that containing about 5% NaCl concentration, and
its capability of surviving through the winter in freezing temperatures.

3. *Brugia malayi*, nocturnally subperiodic

Malayan filariasis found in jungle swamp areas of West Malaysia,
such as in areas along the Pahang River and Perak River, was
reported by Laing *et al.* (1960) to be different from that found in
other open swamp areas of Malaya. The periodicity of microfilariae
was subperiodic. Certain numbers of microfilariae were also found
during the daytime. It has further been confirmed that the parasite
is found among certain wild and domestic animals which serve as
natural reservoirs. Although all the other forms of human filariasis
can theoretically be eradicated by effective treatment of the human
carriers alone, control of this particular type is difficult because of
the presence of animal reservoirs as the source of new infections.

Nocturnally subperiodic Malayan filariasis has been reported by

Rozeboom, Cabrera and others (1964, 1965, 1970) from three regions of the Philippines (Palawan, Sulu Islands and Mindanao). A recent review of the distribution of filariasis in Indonesia by Lie Kian Joe (1970) suggests that there exist both periodic and subperiodic forms in this country. The occurrence of the subperiodic form has been confirmed from Sumatra, Java and Kalimantan. Malayan filariasis reported from North Borneo is also considered to be subperiodic (Barclay, 1965).

Timor filaria

David and Edeson (1965) reported filarial infection among people of Timor (both Portuguese and Indonesian) due to a parasite related to but distinctly different from *Brugia malayi* and it is now tentatively called "Timor filaria" or "*Brugia* (Timor)." Its microfilariae are nocturnally periodic, and differ from those of *B. malayi* in overall length, cephalic space-ratio, and in failure of the sheath to stain with Giemsa. According to the surveys carried out by Ferreira and others (1965, 1966), 533 (5.2%) of 10,200 people examined were microfilaria positive. *Brugia* Timor was present in 84.9%, *W. bancrofti* in 11.3%, and both together in 3.8% of the positive blood films. No adult worms nor intermediate hosts have yet been determined.

Brugia spp. in animals

Besides the occurrence of subperiodic *Brugia malayi* in some wild and domestic animals, several species of *Brugia* have been reported from animals in Asia, such as *B. pahangi* from Malaya, *B. buckleyi* and *B. ceylonensis* from Ceylon. Most of them are indistinguishable from *B. malayi* in microfilariae and mosquito-state larvae, and require examination of adults for identification. Among them, *B. pahangi* was shown to be able to develop in man and produce microfilariae under experimental conditions (Edeson *et al.*, 1960).

SCHISTOSOMIASIS

Human schistosomiasis endemic in Southeast Asia is considered at present to be due to *Schistosoma japonicum* (Katsurada, 1904), and the known intermediate hosts are amphibious snails of the genus *Oncomelania*. Its geographic distribution is more limited than that of filariasis, and endemic areas have been reported only from Japan, continental China, Taiwan, Philippines, Celebes of Indonesia, and Laos-Thai border areas of the Mekong basin. However, the numbers of people

involved and the health hazard to the people in endemic areas are
almost as big as, or may be more serious in schistosomiasis than in
filariasis.

Table 2.   Endemic Areas of *Schistosoma japonicum* in Asia

Country	Endemic area	Population exposed	Intermediate host
Japan	Kofu, Tone, Katayama, Kurume districts	350,000	*Oncomelania nosophora*
Philippines	Leyte, Mindanao, Mindoro, Samar, Luzon Islands	1,550,000	*Oncomelania quadrasi*
China	South of Yangtze River	200,000,000	*Oncomelania hupensis*
Taiwan	Ilan, Changhua provinces	(non-human)	*Oncomelania formosana*
Indonesia	Celebes (Lake Lindu)	10,000 ?	unknown
Thailand	Nakorn Srithammaraj	10,000 ?	unknown
Laos & Cambodia	Mekong River basin	?	unknown

Schistosomiasis in Japan

The disease has a patchy distribution in this country, such as in the
Kofu basin of Yamanashi, the Tone River basin of Kanto District,
Katayama basin of Hiroshima, and the Chikugo River basin of
northern Kyushu. The populations of the endemic areas are estimated to be about 200,000 in Yamanashi, about 20,000 in Hiroshima, and about 52,000 in northern Kyushu. Reviews on the present
status of schistosomiasis in Japan were made by Yokogawa (1970)
and Okabe (1969). Due to the success of various control measures,
especially to the reduction of the population of the snail intermediate
host (as a result of the use of molluscicides and extensive construction
of concrete irrigation ditches), the disease has been remarkably
reduced in all endemic areas. It is anticipated that the snail intermediate host will be eradicated sooner or later from Japan, as has
already been achieved in the Katayama basin. The snail intermediate host in Japan is *Oncomelania hupensis nosophora*.

Schistosomiasis in the Philippines

Schistosomiasis japonica in the Philippines is known from the
islands of Leyte, Mindanao, Samar and Luzon, and about 10% of
the total land with a population of about 300,000 to 500,000 is
estimated to be infected. The prevalence of the disease is especially

serious among people of eastern Leyte. More than half of the people living in this rice-growing area are estimated to be suffering from schistosomiasis. The Philippine government established a Division of schistosomiasis under the Department of Health in 1951, and started extensive research and survey activities aided by WHO and USAID. A comprehensive review of the results was published by Pesigan *et al.* (1958), and by Santos (1969). The snail intermediate host in the Philippines is *O. h. quadrasi.*

Schistosomiasis in mainland China

The largest endemic area of schistosomiasis japonica lies in continental China, and the size of endemic areas as well as the number of people involved are far larger than in the other countries of Asia combined. Visiting Peking in November 1958 as a member of a medical mission to the People's Republic of China, I had the opportunity to discuss the schistosomiasis problem with Prime Minister Mr. Chou En Lai. It was stated by the Chinese authority that the population exposed to the risk of infection is roughly estimated at about 200 million. The areas involved are most of the rice-growing areas along the Yangtse River valley and southern China, and according to the Prime Minister a campaign against schistosomiasis had been launched as an important national policy.

Details of the results of surveys and control activities carried out by Chinese authorities and scientists have remained inaccessible to us during the past ten years. However, an excellent review was published recently by Tien-Hsi Cheng (1971) in the *American Journal of Tropical Medicine and Hygiene,* referring to schistosomiasis research and control programs since 1949 in mainland China. As a result of more than half a century of neglect of public health in this country, central China was ravaged by schistosomiasis when the campaign started in 1949. The surveys showed that the endemic areas were distributed in at least 11 provinces comprising 324 districts, and that about 10.5 million people had schistosomiasis and another 100 million were exposed constantly to the danger of infection. Also, 1.5 million cattle were infected. The national campaign against schistosomiasis utilized abundant manpower to destroy the habitats of *Oncomelania hupensis* by cleaning irrigation ditches and streams and by reclaiming lands *via* earth fills. The snail intermediate host in mainland China is *O. hupensis hupensis.*

Schistosomiasis in Taiwan

A parasite morphologically indistinguishable from *Schistosoma japonicum* was found among wild and domestic animals in Changhua and Ilan. However, no human infection has ever been found among the inhabitants of the same areas. Results of human experiments with cercariae obtained from the snail intermediate host, *O. formosana*, carried out by Hsü *et al.* (1965) also suggest that the parasite is not adapted for development in human beings. Another species of the snail intermediate host, *O. chiui*, was found in the Ali-lao district near Taipei, and was shown experimentally to be adapted for the development of various human strains of *S. japonicum*, but no natural infection of snails and animals has been detected. Fan and Khaw (1969) published a review of the schistosomiasis problem of Taiwan.

Schistosomiasis in Indonesia

An endemic area of schistosomiasis was reported from villages near Lindu Lake, middle Celebes, by Brug and Tesch (1937). This and later surveys carried out before the World War II by Dutch workers (Muller and Tesch, 1937; Bonne, *et al.*, 1940, 1942) have shown that the disease is highly prevalent among people and animals of this area. The snail intermediate host still remains unknown.

Schistosomiasis in Laos, Thailand and Cambodia

A severe case of infection with schistosomes was diagnosed in 1957 in Paris by liver biopsy of a student from Laos. The patient was native to an island on the Mekong near the Thai and Cambodian border. A series of surveys sponsored by WHO were carried out in these areas, and an endemic area was discovered in 1966 by Iijima and Garcia on Khong Island, southern Laos. Of 547 stool samples examined, 8.5% were positive for schistosome eggs. A review was published by Pathammavong (1969), and the first report by Iijima *et al.* (1971) appeared in the *Japanese Journal of Parasitology*.

In Thailand, Chaiyaporn, *et al.*, (1959) reported a case of schistosomiaisis in a farmer in Nakorn Srithammaraj Province, southern Thailand near the West Malaysian border. Harinasuta and Kruatrachue (1960, 1962) carried out epidemiological surveys of this area and found 50 egg-positive cases among 2,667 people. They also reported another endemic area in the Mekong Basin near the Laos border, where two positive cases were detected among 400 people of Ubol Province.

In Cambodia also, a case of schistosomiasis was reported by Aubebaud *et al.*, (1968) from the Mekong Basin, and an endemic focus was discovered from Kratie District. Further epidemiological studies are in progress by Tournier *et al.* (1970).

In all of these endemic areas, previous efforts to determine the snail intermediate host have been unsuccessful, and no *Oncomelania* snails have ever been discovered. Sornmani (1969) carried out experimental infection of four known intermediate hosts of *S. japonicum* (*O. nosophora, O. hupensis, O. formosana* and *O. quadrasi*) with miracidia hatched from human feces, but no development of cercariae was seen in these snails with the Thai strain of *Schistosoma*.

REFERENCES

Among large numbers of papers published in the past referring to the epidemiology of filariasis and schistosomiasis in the Asiatic-Pacific region, the following selected papers are cited for the convenience of workers further interested in this field. These are among the principal references utilized in compiling this manuscript, though there are a number of papers coming before for which references are included. The papers used in compiling the present review were collected mainly by reviewing the *Tropical Diseases Bulletin* and also by personal communication with workers in these fields throughout the world. I am especially indebted to Dr. C. P. Ramachandran for providing information through his mimeographed manuscript on the epidemiology of filariasis in Asia.

"FILARIASIS"

Abdulcader, M. H. M. and Sasa, M. (1966). Epidemiology and control of bancroftian filariasis in Ceylon. *Japan. J. Exp. Med.*, **36**, 609.

Abdulcader, M. H. M. (1967). Present status of *Brugia malayi* infection in Ceylon. *J. Trop. Med. & Hyg.*, **70**, 199.

Barclay, R. (1965). Filariasis in South-West Sabah. *Ann. Trop. Med. & Parasit.*, **59**, 340.

Barclay, R. (1969). Filariasis in Sabah, East Malaysia. *Ann. Trop. Med. & Parasit.*, **63**, 473.

Barry, C. *et al.* (1971). Endemic filariasis in Thakurgaon, East Pakistan. *Amer. J. Trop. Med. Y Hyg.*, **20**, 592.

Brug, S. L. (1927). *Filaria malayi* n.sp. parasitic in man in the Malay archipelago. Trans. of the F.E.A.T.M. 7th Congr., India, **3**, 279.

Buckley, J. J. C. and Edeson, J. F. B. (1956). On the adult morphology of *Wuchereria* sp. (*malayi* ?) from a monkey (*Macaca irus*) and from cats in Malaya, and on *Wuchereria pahangi* n.sp. from a dog and cat. *J. Helminth.*, **30**, 1.

Buckley, J. J. C. (1960). On *Brugia* gen. nov. for *Wuchereria* spp. of the "*malayi*" group i.e. *W. malayi* (Brug, 1927), *W. pahangi* Buckley and Edeson, 1956, *W. patei* Buckley,

Nelson and Heisch, 1958. *Ann. Trop. Med. & Parasit.*, **54**, 75.

Burnett, G. F. (1960). Filariasis research in Fiji, 1957–9, under Colonial Development and Welfare Schemes 823 and 829. Rep. of the Secretary of State for the Colonies. 157 pp.

Cabrera, B. D. and Tubangui, M. (1951). Studies on filariasis in the Philippines. III. *Aedes (Finlaya) poicilius* (Theobald), the mosquito intermediate host of *Wuchereria bancrofti* in the Bicol region. *Acta Med. Phil.*, **7**, 221.

Cabrera, B. D. and Rozeboom, L. E. (1965). The periodicity characters of the filaria parasites of man in the Republic of the Philippines. *Amer. J. Epidemiol.*, **81**, 192.

Caberera, B. D. and Tamondong, C. T. (1966). Bancroftian and Malayan filariasis in Palawan. Extent and distribution. *Acta Med. Phil.*, **3**, 20.

Cabrera, B. D. and Tamondong, C. (1966). Filariasis survey in Jolo, Sulu. *Acta Med. Phil.*, **3**, 86.

Cabrera, B. D. and Cruz, I. (1968).The second endemic focus for Malayan filariasis in the Republic of the Philippines. *Acta Med. Phil.*, **5**, 1.

Cabrera, B. D. (1968). Determination of mosquito vector of filariasis in southern Sulu. *J. Phil. Med. Assoc.*, **44**, 117.

Cabrera, B. D. and Tamondong, C. T. (1970). Filariasis studies in Mindanao Island. *J. Phil. Med. Assoc.*, **46**, 74.

Cabrera, B. D. (1970). *Brugia malayi* vector determination in Bunawan, Agusan, the third endemic focus for Malayan filariasis in the Philippines. *Southeast Asian J. Trop. Med. & Pub. Hlth.*, **1**, 496.

Chen, K. C. (1948). A note on the filaria survey in Fukien province. *Lingnan Sci. J.*, **22**, 85.

Ciferri, F., *et al.* (1968). A filariasis control program in American Samoa. *Amer. J. Trop. Med. & Hyg.*, **18**, 369.

Colwell, E. J. *et al.* (1970). Epidemiologic and serologic investigations of filariasis in indigenous populations and American soldiers in South Vietnam. *Amer. J. Trop. Med. & Hyg.*, **19**, 227.

David, H. L. and Edeson, J. F. B. (1965). Filariasis in Portuguese Timor, with observations on a new microfilaria found in man. *Ann. Trop. Med. & Parasit.*, **59**, 193.

de Meillon, B. *et al.* (1967). Reports from WHO Filariasis Research Unit, Rangoon. *Bull. Wld Hlth Org.*, **36**, 1–100.

Demos, E. A., *et al.* (1954). Malaria and filariasis investigation in Pescadores (Peng-Hu) Islands of Taiwan, Republic of China. *J. Formosan Med. Assoc.*, **53**, 541.

Dissanaike, A. S. and Paramananthan, D. C. (1961). On *Brugia* (*Brugiella* subgen. nov.) *buckleyi* n. sp. from the heart and blood vessels of the Ceylon hare. *J. Helminth.*, **35**, 209.

Dissanaike, A. S. (1969). Control of filariasis in Ceylon. Proc. Seminar on Filariasis & Immun. Parasitic Inf. & Lab. Meeting, Singapore—1968, pp. 149–161.

Dissanaike, A. S. (1969). The status of research and study of filariasis in Ceylon. Proc. Seminar on Filariasis & Immun. Parasitic Inf. & Lab. Meeting, Singapore—1968, pp. 210–217.

Dunn, F. L. and Ramachandran, C. P. (1969). South-East Asian filarioids with special reference to those normally parasitic in vertebrates other than man. Proc. Seminar on Filariasis & Immun. Parasitic Inf. & Lab. Meeting, Singapore—1968, pp. 194–209.

Edeson, J. F. B., Wilson, T., Wharton, R. H. and Laing, A. B. G. (1960).   Experimental transmission of *Brugia malayi* and *B. pahangi* to man. *Trans. Roy. Soc. Trop. Med. & Parasit.*, **57**, 75.

Edeson, J. F. B. (1962).   The epidemiology and treatment of infection due to *Brugia malayi.*, *Bull. Wld Hlth Org.*, **27**, 529.

Edeson, J. F. B. and Wilson, T. (1964).   The epidemiology of filariasis due to *Wuchereria bancrofti* and *Brugia malayi.*, *Annual Rev. Entomology*, **9**, 245.

Estrada, J. P. and Basio, D. G. (1965).   Filariasis in the Philippines. *J. Phil. Med. Assoc.*, **41**, 100.

Fan, P. C. and Hsu, J. (1954).   Filariasis in Free China. Pt. I. Incidence in Taiwan, Peng-Hu (Pescadores) and Kinmen (Quemoy). *Chin, Med. J.*, Taipei, **1**, 77.

Fan, P. C. and Hsu, J. (1955).   Filariasis in Free China. Pt. II. Incidence in Taiwan Chinese. *Chin. Med. J.*, Taipei, **2**, 151.

Fan, P. C. and Hsu, J. (1957).   Filariasis in Free China. Pt. III. Incidence in Penghu Chinese. *Chin. Med. J.*, Taipei, **4**, 35.

Fan, P. C. and Hsu, J. (1957).   Filariasis in Free China. Pt. IV. Incidence in Kinmen Chinese. *Chin. Med. J.*, Taipei, **4**, 81.

Feng, L. C. (1931).   Filariasis in China with special reference to its distribution and transmission. *Chin. Med. J.*, **17**, 464.

Ferreira, F. S. C., Gunha, C. A. C. L., Vieira, R. A. and Matias, M. F. (1965).   Lymphatic filariasis in Portuguese Timor. I. General aspect of infection by *Brugia* (Timor). *Anais Inst. Med. Trop.*, **22**, **75**.

Hairston, N. G. and Jachowski, L. A., Jr. (1968).   Analysis of the *Wuchereria bancrofti* population in the people of American Samoa. *Bull. Wld Hlth Org.*, **38**, 29.

Harinasuta, C. *et al.* (1970a).   Studies on Malayan filariasis in Thailand. *Southeast Asian J. Trop. Med. & Pub. Hlth.*, **1**, 29.

Harinasuta, C. *et al.* (1970b).   Observations on the six-year results of the pilot project for the control of Malayan filariasis in Thailand. *Southeast Asian J. Trop. Med. & Pub. Hlth.*, **1**, 205.

Harinasuta, C. *et al.* (1970c).   Bancroftian filariasis in Thailand, a new endemic area. *Southeast Asian J. Trop. Med. & Pub. Hlth.*, **1**, 233.

Hawking, F. (1962).   A review of progress in the chemotherapy and control of filariasis since 1955. *Bull. Wld Hlth Org.*, **27**, 555.

Hu, M. K., *et al.* (1937).   A brief survey of filariasis in Foochow and Futsing region, South China. *Chin. Med. J.*, **52**, 571.

Iyenger, M. O. T. (1952).   Filariasis in the Maldive Islands. *Bull. Wld Hlth Org.*, **7**, 375.

Jachowski, L. A., Jr. and Otto, G. F. (1955).   Filariasis in American Samoa. VI. Prevalence of microfilaremia in the human population. *Amer. J. Hy.*, **61**, 334.

Jayewardene, L. G. (1962).   On two filarial parasites from dogs in Ceylon, *Brugia ceylonensis* and *Dipetalonema* sp. inq. *J. Helminth.*, **36**, 269.

Joseph, G. and Prasad, B. G. (1967).   An epidemiological study of filariasis in the coastal belt of Kerala State. *Indian J. med. Res.*, **55**, 1259.

Kessel, J. F. (1957).   An effective programme for the control of filariasis in Tahiti. *Bull. Wld Hlth Org.*, **16**, 633.

Kessel, J. F. (1960).   Non-periodic bancroftian filariasis. *Ind. J. Malariol.*, **14**, 509.

Kessel, J. F. and Massal, E. (1962).   Control of bancroftian filariasis in the Pacific. *Bull. Wld Hlth Org.*, **27**, 543.

Kessel, J. F. (1966).   Filariasis as a World Problem. *Mosquito News*, **26**, 490.

Laigret, J., *et al.* (1965).   La lutte contre la filariose lymphatique aperiodique en Polynesie Française. *Bull. Soc. Path. Exot.*, **58**, 895.

Laing, A. B. G. (1960).   A review of recent research on filariasis in Malaya. *Indian J. Malariol.*, **14**, 391.

Lee, K. T. (1961).   Malayan filariasis. The first report on incidence and distribution among children in Cheju-Do island. *Bull. National Inst. Hlth, ROK.*, **4**, 107.

Lee, K. T., *et al.* (1964).   Malayan filariasis. 2nd report: Epidemiological investigations on filariasis due to *Brugia malayi* in the residents of southern Cheju-Do island. *J. Korean Med. Assoc.*, **7**, 657.

Lie Kian Joe, *et al.* (1960).   *Wuchereria bancrofti* infection in Djakarta, Indonesia. A study of some factors influencing its transmission. *Indian J. Malariol.*, **14**, 339.

Lie Kian Joe (1970).   The distribution of filariasis in Indonesia. *Southeast Asian J. Trop. Med. & Pub. Hlth.*, **1**, 366.

Mackerras, M. J. (1958).   The decline of filariasis in Queensland. *Med. J. Australia*, **9**, 3.

Marshall, C. L. and Yasukawa, K. (1966).   Control of bancroftian filariasis in the Ryukyu Islands: Preliminary results of mass administration of diethylcarbamazine. *Amer. J. Trop. Med. & Hyg.*, **15**, Pt. 1, 934.

Mataika, U. J. (1965).   Filariasis in the Solomon Islands. A survey on Guadalcanal and Florida Islands. Report to WHO Seminar on Filariasis, Manila, 6 pp.

McMillan, B. (1967).   Is filariasis endemic in the Northern Territory of Australia? *Med. J. Australia*, **2**, 243.

Nair, C. P. (1966).   Filaria survey of Palghat Town, Kerala State. *Bull. Indian Soc. Mal. & Comm. Dis.*, **3**, 198.

Nair, C. P. and Bhatnagar, V. N. (1968).   Filariasis in Kerala, south India. Filarial survey of Trichur town. *Antiseptic*, **65**, 235.

Oemijati, S. and Liem Kiat Tjoen (1966).   Filariasis in Timor. Proc. 11th Pacific Sci. Congr. **8**, 5.

Paik, Y. H., *et al.* (1957).   Epidemiological survey on filariasis in Nonsan area. *Korean Med. J.*, **2**, 1175.

Raghavan, N. G. S. (1957).   Epidemiology of filariasis in India. *Bull. Wld Hlth Org.*, **16**, 553.

Raghavan, N. G. S. (1961).   The vectors of human infections by *Wuchereria* species in endemic areas and their biology. *Bull. Wld Hlth Org.*, **24**, 177.

Ramachandran, C. P., Hoo, C. C. and Omar, A. H. (1964).   Filariasis among aborigines and Malays living close to Kuala Lumpur. *Med. J. Malaya*, **18**, 193.

Ramachandran, C. P. (1970).   Filariasis in Ulu Trengganu, West Malaysia: Parasitological and entomological observations. *Southeast Asian J. Trop. Med. & Pub. Hlth.*, 505.

Ramakrishnan, S. P. *et al.* (1960).   National filaria control programme in India. A review. *Indian J. Malariol.*, **14**, 457.

Ramalingam, S. and Belkin, N. J. (1964).   Vectors of subperiodic bancroftian filariasis in the Samoan-Tonga area. *Nature*, **201**, 105.

Ramalingam, S. (1968).   The epidemiology of filarial transmission in Samoa and Tonga. *Ann. Trop. Med. & Parasit.*, **62**, 305.

Ramalingam, S., *et al.* (1969).   The vectors of *Wuchereria bancrofti* and *Brugia malayi* in

South-East Asia. Proc. Seminar on Filariasis & Immun. Parasitic Inf. & Lab. Meeting, Singapore—1968, pp. 172–193.

Rozeboom, L. E. and Cabrera, B. D. (1956).   Filariasis in the Philippine Islands. *Amer. J. Hyg.*, **63**, 140.

Rozeboom, L. E. and Cabrera, B. D. (1963).   Transmission of filariasis in the Philippine Islands by *Anopheles minimum flavirostris* Ludlow. *Nature*, **200**, 915.

Rozeboom, L. E. and Cabrera, B. D. (1964).   Filariasis in Mountain Province, Luzon, Republic of the Philippines. *J. Med. Entom.*, **1**, 18.

Rozeboom, L. E. and Cabrera, B. D. (1965).   Filariasis caused by *Brugia malayi* in the Republic of the Philippines. *Amer. J. Epidemiol.*, **81**, 200.

Rozeboom, L. E. and Cabrera, B. D. (1965).   Filariasis caused by *Wuchereria bancrofti* in Palawan, Republic of the Philippines. *Amer. J. Epidemiol.*, **81**, 216.

Rozeboom, L. E. and Cabrera, B. D. (1966).   Filariasis in the Republic of the Philippines: Epidemiology and possible origins. *Acta Med. Phil.*, **3**, 112.

Samarawickerema, W. A. (1970).   A study of the age-composition of natural populations of *Culex pipiens fatigans* in relation to the transmission of filariasis due to *Wuchereria bancrofti* (Cobbold) in Ceylon. *Bull. Wld Hlth Org.*, **37**, 117.

Sasa, M. (1962).   Distribution of bancroftian filariasis in Japan. In "Advances in Parasitology in Japan," **2**, 1 Meguro Kiseichukan, Tokyo.

Sasa, M., *et al.* (1966).   Comparative studies on some morphological and physiological characters of the *Culex pipiens* complex of Japan and southern Asia. *Japan. J. Exp. Med.*, **37**, 477.

Sasa, M. (1966).   Epidemiology of human filariasis in Japan. Progress in Medical Parasitology in Japan, **3**, 3.

Sasa, M. (1967).   Microfilaria survey methods and analysis of survey data in filariasis control programmes. *Bull. Wld Hlth Org.*, **37**, 629.

Sasa, M. (1970).   "On the progress of filariasis control programme in Okinawa" *Nettai*, **5**, 89. (in Japanese)

Sasa, M., *et al.* (1970).   The filariasis control programmes in Japan and their evaluation by means of the microfilaria survey data. Recent Advances in Researches on Filariasis and Schistosomiasis in Japan, 3–72; Univ. Tokyo Press.

Senoo, T. and Lincicome, D. R. (1951).   Malayan filariasis incidence and distribution in southern Korea. *U.S.A.F. Med. J.*, **2**, 1183.

Sery, V., *et al.* (1961).   La filariose au Vietnam du Nord. *Ceskoslov. Parasit.* (Prague), **8**, 391.

Soh, Chin-Thack (1965).   "Filariasis in Korea", in "Review of Parasites in Korea, 23–31; Yonsei Univ. Med. College, Seoul.

Song, J. S. and Lee, K. T. (1964).   Report on filariasis at Danyang district, Choong-chung-Fukdo. *Korean J. Parasit.*, **2**, 125.

Stoll, N. R. (1947).   This wormy world. *J. Parasit.*, **33**, 1.

South Pacific Commission (1953).   Filariasis in the Pacific. 108 pp., Noumea; (various authors, proceedings of a conference at Papeete, Tahiti, 1951).

Tanaka, S. (1937).   Investigation and clinical observations on microfilariae among Formosan Chinese in Hoko Islands (Pescadores). *J. Formosan Med. Assoc.*, **36**, 815.

Wharton, R. H. (1960).   Studies on filariasis in Malaya: Field and laboratory investigations of the vector of a rural strain of *Wuchereria bancrofti.*, *Ann. Trop. Med. & Parasit.*, **54**, 78.

Wharton, R. H. (1962). The biology of *Mansonia* mosquitoes in relation to the transmission of filariasis in Malaya. Bull. No. 11, Inst. Med. Res. Malaya, 114 pp.

Wilson, T. (1969). An example of filariasis control from West Malaysia. *Bull. Wld Hlth Org.*, **41**, 324.

Wolfe, M. S. and Aslamkan, M. (1968). Ecology of filariasis in East Pakistan. Trans. 8th Intern. Congr. Trop. Med. & Malaria, pp. 113–114 (Teheran)

Wolfe, M. S. and Aslamkan, M. (1969). Filariasis survey in Karachi. *Trans. Royal Soc. Trop Med. & Hyg.*, **63**, 147.

Wolfe, M. S. and Aslamkan, M. (1971). Filariasis in East Pakistan. *Trans. Roy. Soc. Trop. Med. & Hyg.*, **65**, 63.

World Health Organization (1967). WHO Expert Committee on Filariasis, Second Report; WHO Tech. Rep. Ser. No. 359, 47 pp.

World Health Organization (1968). Filariasis; in Wld Hlth Statist. Rep. **21**, 576.

World Health Organization/South Pacific Commission (1968). Second WHO/SPO Joint Seminar on Filariasis, Apia, Western Samoa; 44 Mim. pages, WPR/350/68.

Yokogawa, S. *et al.* (1939). Epidemiological investigation on *Wuchereria bancrofti* in the Hoko Islands (Pescadores). *J. Formosan Med. Assoc.*, **38**, 1939. (in Japanese)

Zulueta, J. de (1957). Observations on filariasis in Sarawak and Brunei. *Bull. Wld Hlth Org.*, **16**, 699.

"SCHISTOSOMIASIS"

Audebaud, G. *et al.* (1968). Premier cas de bilharziose humaine observé au Cambodge (Région de Kratie). *Bull. Soc. Path. Exot.*, **61**, 778.

Barbier, M. (1966). Determination d'un foyer de bilharziose arterio-veineuse au Sud-Laos (Province de Sithadone). *Bull. Soc. Path. Exot.*, **59**, 974.

Bonne, C. and Sandground, J. H. (1940). *Bilharzia japonicum* aan het Lindumeer. *Gen. Tijdschr. Ned. Indie*, **80**, 477.

Bonne, C. *et al.* (1942). Voortgezet bilharzia onderzoek in Celebes. *Gen. Tijdschr. Ned. Indie*, **82**, 21.

Brug, S. L. and Tesch, J. W. (1937). Parasitaire wormen aan het Lindumeer. *Gen. Tijdschr. Ned. Indie*, **77**, 2151.

Chaiyaporn, V. *et al*, (1959). The first case of *Schistosomiasis japonicum* in Thailand. *J. Med. Assoc. Thailand*, **42**, 328.

Cheng, Tien-Hsi (1971). Schistosomiasis in Mainland China. A review of research and control programs since 1940. *Amer. J. Trop. Med. & Hyg.*, **20**, 26.

Chi, L. W. *et al.* (1971). Susceptibility of *Oncomelania* hybrid snails to various geographic strains of *Schistosoma japonicum*. *Amer. J. Trop. Med. & Hyg.*, **20**, 89.

Chiu, J. K. (1965). *Tricula chiui*: a new snail host for Formosan strain of *S. japonicum*. *J. Parasit.*, **51**, 206.

Chiu, J. K. (1967). Susceptibility of *O. hupensis chiui* to infection with *S. japonicum*. *Malacologia*, **6**, 145.

Chiu, J. K. (1968). Cercaria production of geographic strains of *Schistosoma japonicum* in *Oncomelania hupensis chiui*. *J. Formosan Med. Assoc.*, **76**, 259.

Davis, G. M. (1969). *Oncomelania* and the transmission of *Schistosoma japonicum*: A brief review. *Proc. 4th S-E Asian Seminar, pp. 93–103.

Fan, P. C. and Khaw, O. K. (1969). Schistosomiasis japonica in Taiwan: A review. *Proc. 4th S-E Asian Seminar, pp. 17–47; also in "*Chin. Med. J.* Taipei 16:100–

130".

Faust, E. C. and Meleny, H. E. (1924). Schistosomiasis japonica. *Amer. J. Hyg. Mon. Ser. No.*, **3**, 1.

Garcia, E. Y. (1967). *Schistosoma philippinensis*, a new species of human schistosome in the Philippines. *Helminthologia*, **8**, 147.

Harinasuta, C. and Kruatrachue, M. (1960). Schistosomiasis in Thailand. *Trans. Roy. Soc. Trop. Med. & Hyg.*, **54**, 280.

Harinasuta, C. and Kruatrachue, M. (1962). The first recognized endemic area of Bilharziasis in Thailand. *Ann. Trop. Med. & Parasit.*, **56**, 314.

Harinasuta, C. and Sornmani, S. (1969). Non-human schistosomiasis in southern Asia: A review. *Proc. 4th S-E Asian Seminar, pp. 111–115.

Hsü, H. F. and Hsü Li, S. Y. (1962). *Schistosoma japonicum* in Formosa. A critical review. *Exp. Parasit.*, **12**, 459.

Hsü, H. F. and Hsü Li, S. Y. (1967). The race complex of *O. formosana* in Taiwan, China. *Z. Tropenmed. & Parasit.*, **18**, 417.

Hsü, H. F. and Hsü Li, S. Y. (1968). The strain complex of *S. japonicum* in Taiwan, China. *Z. Tropenmed. & Parasit.*, **19**, 43.

Iijima, T., *et al.* (1971). Studies on schistosomiasis in the Mekong Basin. I. Morphological observation on the schistosomes and detection of their reservoir hosts. *Japan. J. Parasit.*, **20**, 24.

Khaw, O. K. and Fan, P. C. (1966). Schistosomiasis japonica in Taiwan. *Chin. Med. J., Taipei*, **13**, 128.

Komiya, Y. (1960). Study and application of molluscicides in Japan. *Bull. Wld Hlth Org.*, **25**, 573.

Komiya, Y. (1965). Cementing ditches of the habitat of *Oncomelania nosophora*, the intermediate host of *Schistosoma japonicum*, as a preventive measure of schistosomiasis. A review. *Jap. J. Med. Sci. Biol.*, **18**, 275.

Kunz, R. E. (1965). Zoophilic schistosomiasis with a report of a new locality on Taiwan. *J. Formosan Med. Assoc.*, **64**, 649.

Lee, H. F. and Wykoff, D. E. (1966). Schistosomes from wild rats in Thailand. *J. Parasit.*, **52**, 323.

Muller, H. and Tesch, J. W. (1937). Autochtone infectie met *Schistosoma japonicum* op Celebes. *Gen. Tijdschr. Ned. Indie*, **77**, 2143.

Oemijati, S. (1969). Schistosomiasis in Indonesia: A review. *Proc. 4th S-E Asian Seminar, pp. 59–63.

Okabe, K. (1964). Biology and epidemiology of *Schistosoma japonicum* and schistosomiasis. Progress of Medical Parasitology in Japan, **1**, 185.

Okabe, K. (1969). Schistosomiasis japonica in Japan: A review. *Proc. 4th S-E Asian Seminar. pp. 9–13.

Okabe, K. (1971). The epidemiology and preventive measures of *Schistosoma japonicum*. *Japan. J. Trop. Med.*, **11**, 1.

Pathammavong, O. (1969). Schistosomiasis in Laos. *Proc. 4th S-E. Asian Seminar pp. 65–69.

Pesigan, T. P. *et al.* (1958). Studies on *Schistosoma japonicum* infection in the Philippines. *Bull. Wld Hlth Org.*, **18**, 345.

Santos, A. T., Jr. (1969). Schistosomiasis control in the Philippines: A review. *Proc. 4th S-E. Asian Seminar, pp. 1–7.

Santos, A. T. *et al.* (1969). A report of two schistosomiasis endemic municipalities in northwestern Leyte. *J. Phil. Med. Assoc.*, **45**, 690.

Sornmani, S. (1969). Schistosomiasis in Thailand: A review. *Proc. 4th S-E Asian Seminar, 71–82.

Tournier-Lasserve, C., Jolly, M. *et al.* (1970). Existence au Cambodge d'un foyer de bilharziose humaine, dans la region de Kratie. I. Étude des trois premiers cas cliniques. II. Enquete epidemiologique—resultats preliminaires. *Med. Trop.*, **30**, 451; 462.

Wagner, E. D. and Chi, L. W. (1959). Species crossing in *Oncomelania Amer. J. Trop. Med. & Hyg.*, **8**, 195.

Warren, K. S. and Newill, V. A. (1967). Schistosomiasis. A bibliography of world's literature from 1952 to 1962. Vol. 1 & 2, 598 & 395 pp. Western Reserve Univ. Press, Cleveland.

World Health Organization (1967). Epidemiology and control of schistosomiasis. Report of a WHO Expert Committee. *WHO Tech. Rep. Ser.*, No. 372, 33 pp.

World Health Organization (1969). Schistosomiasis, in *WHO Statist. Rep.*, **22**(3), 233–247.

Wright, W. H. (1950). Bilharziasis as a public-health problem in the Pacific. *Bull. Wld Hlth Org.*, **2**, 581.

Yasuraoka, K. (1969). Snail vectors in schistosomiasis japonica. *Proc. 4th S-E. Asian Seminar. pp. 83–91.

Yasuraoka, K. (1969). Control of schistosomiasis japonica. *Proc. S-E Asian Seminar, pp. 149–156.

Yokogawa, M. (1970). Schistosomiasis in Japan. in "Recent Advances in Researches on Filariasis and Schistosomiasis in Japan, pp. 231–255, Univ. Tokyo Press.

Yuan, H. C. (1958). A preliminary study on the susceptibility of geographic strains of *Oncomelania hupensis* to geographic strains of *Schistosoma japonicum* from 6 different provinces in China. *Chin. Med. J.*, Peking, **77**, 575.

* Proceedings of the 4th Southeast Asian Seminar on Parasitology and Tropical Medicine; schistosomiasis and other snail-transmitted helminthiasis, Manila—1969; SEAMEC-TROPMED, Bangkok

Eradication Experiment of Bancroftian Filariasis in the Control of Vector Mosquitoes in Nagate Village, Nagasaki Prefecture*

N. Omori,** Y. Wada and T. Oda

*Department of Medical Zoology, Nagasaki University
School of Medicine, Nagasaki, Japan*

INTRODUCTION

Since bancroftian filariasis caused by *Wuchereria bancrofti* is transmitted from man to man only by vector mosquitoes, it is supposed that without vector mosquitoes no transmission will occur and adult filariae in an infected person will die some years after infection. Investigations along this line were thought to be very useful for understanding the epidemiology of bancroftian filariasis and therefore a filariasis eradication experiment involving only the control of vector mosquitoes was planned from 1962 at Nagate Village, Nagasaki Prefecture, southern Japan. In the experiment, persons were not to be treated with drugs. In 1961, the year before the start of mosquito control, microfilarial prevalence in all persons of the village was 14.0%, but it decreased steadily year by year and was found to be 7.9% in 1965 (Wada, 1966b). A yearly decrease was steadily observed after that, and microfilarial prevalence in 1970 was only 0.5 %. In the present paper successful reduction of filariasis endemicity will be described in relation to the control of vector mosquitoes as seen by the results gathered from 1961 to 1970. The average period of time that infected persons remain positive for microfilaremia will be discussed on the basis of the state of disappearance of microfilariae in infected individuals.

---

* Contribution No. 200 from the Department of Medical Zoology, Nagasaki University School of Medicine

** Present address: Department of Parasitology, School of Medicine, Teikyo University, Tokyo

[21]

PLACE AND METHODS

Nagate Village, where the present experiment was carried out, is situated near the seacoast on Fukue Island, Nagasaki Prefecture, southern Japan. The villagers grow sweet potatoes and also raise cattle, and there are no paddy-fields. In 1961 when we started to examine the status of filariasis and the abundance and natural infection of mosquitoes, there were 126 houses in which 577 persons lived. There were many favorable breeding places such as ditches and foul water pits for *Culex pipiens pallens*, the most important vector of bancroftian filariasis in Japan (Omori, 1962). The secondary but much less important vector of the disease is *Aedes togoi* which breeds in rock pools on the seacoast. The latter, however, were very few in number around this village (Wada, 1966a). Therefore, mosquito control was conducted particularly against *C. p. pallens*.

From 1962 to 1970, residual spraying of insecticides was carried out on inside walls and ceilings of all dwellings and cowsheds once a year, and repeated larvicide applications given against all possible breeding places of *C. p. pallens* during the breeding seasons, as shown in Table 1. The residual spraying was made at a rate of 50 ml per m² by using a 5 % DDT emulsion in 1962, and thereafter a 0.5 % diazinon emulsion. A 5 % diazinon emulsion concentrate was applied as larvicide at a rate of about 1 ppm to the estimated water volume.

Table 1.   Outlines of Control Works against the Vector Mosquito of Bancroftian Filariasis, *C. p. pallens*, in Nagate Village.

Year	Residual spraying			Larvicide application			
	Insecticide	Date	Volume (liters) per house	Insecticide	Period	Times	Total volume (liters)
1962	5% DDT E.	Jun. 6– 7	7.5	5% diaz. E.C.	Jul. 20–Oct. 18	14	16.3
1963	0.5% diaz. E.	Jun. 12–13	7.2	5% diaz. E.C.	Jun. 4–Oct. 28	22	22.4
1964	0.5% diaz. E.	Jun. 15–16	8.2	5% diaz. E.C.	May 16–Oct. 29	25	24.0
1965	0.5% diaz. E.	Jun. 18–19	6.7	5% diaz. E.C.	Jun. 9–Oct. 27	21	24.8
1966	0.5% diaz. E.	Jun. 9–10	7.9	5% diaz. E.C.	May 22–Oct. 10	21	21.1
1967	0.5% diaz. E.	Jun. 20–21	7.4	5% diaz. E.C.	May 29–Oct. 9	20	19.7
1968	0.5% diaz. E.	Jun. 26–27	7.8	5% diaz. E.C.	May 10–Oct. 25	25	28.3
1969	0.5% diaz. E.	Jun. 27	7.0	5% diaz. E.C.	May 12–Oct. 20	24	26.6
1970	0.5% diaz. E.	Jun. 26	7.5	5% diaz. E.C.	May 16–Oct. 24	24	24.9

E.: Emulsion.   E.C.: Emulsion concentrate.   diaz.: diazinon

After 1961, all persons over one year of age in Nagate Village were examined annually for microfilariae. Sixty mm³ of blood was taken on two or three glass slides from an earlobe of each person. The blood film on the slide was dried, stained by Giemsa's solution, and examined microscopically for microfilariae.

DECREASE IN THE DENSITY OF *C. p. pallens*

The seasonal prevalence of *C. p. pallens* females from 1961 to 1970 is given in Fig. 1. In 1961, when mosquito control had not yet been started, the vector mosquito increased in number from the beginning of June, reached a peak in July, decreased thereafter, and the number became very small after October. In 1962 the start of antilarval measures was postponed until July, one and one-half months after

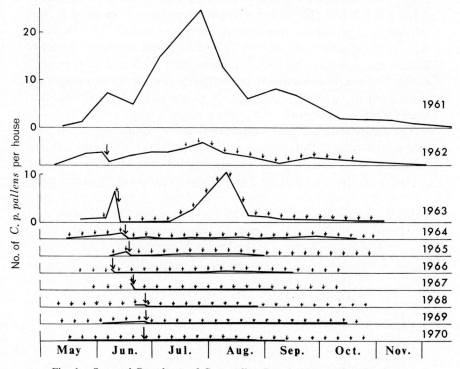

Fig. 1. Seasonal Prevalence of *C. p. pallens* Females Collected in Houses at Nagate Village in the Ten Years from 1961 to 1970, Under Controlled Conditions by Residual Spraying (Large Arrow) and Larvicide Applications (Small Arrows) from 1962 (See Table 1).

the residual spraying, and in 1963 some new breeding places appeared unexpectedly because of a change in the waterways. For these reasons, a number of *C. p. pallens* emerged in both those years, but the density through the years was much lower than in 1961. In 1964 and thereafter, the vector mosquito was nearly completely controlled.

REDUCTION OF PREVALENCE AND DENSITY OF MICROFILARIAE

The reduction of microfilarial prevalence and density in 60 mm^3 blood of all persons in the village is given in Table 2. In 1961 the number of persons found positive for microfilariae was 81 out of 577 villagers, the positive rate having been 14.0 %; the mean number of microfilariae for positives was 79.1 and for all persons, 11.11. After 1962, when the vector mosquito control was in process, the microfilarial prevalence and density decreased steadily year by year. In 1970 the positive rate was 0.5 % and the mean numbers of microfilariae for positives and for all persons were 12.0 and 0.06 respectively. The yearly reduction in microfilarial prevalence and density is considered to be chiefly attributable to the natural death of adult filaria worms in patients.

The above data are based on examinations conducted on all persons in the village. But, change in the population of Nagate Village, including microfilarial positives, occurred during the experimental period from 1961 to 1970. In Table 3, the populations between 1961

Table 2. Reduction of Microfilarial Prevalence and Density in 60 mm^3 Blood of All Persons in Nagate Village during the Ten Years of Continuous Control of the Vector Mosquito after 1961.

Year	1961	1962	1963	1964	1965	1966	1967	1968	1969	1970
No. of persons examined (A)	577	571	567	541	493	515	491	441	447	430
No. of mf. positives (B)	81	71	62	53	39	31	20	9	5	2
% mf. positives $100 \times (B)/(A)$	14.0	12.4	10.9	9.8	7.9	6.0	4.1	2.0	1.1	0.5
Total No. of mf. (C)	6,408	4,794	3,851	1,761	1,057	889	402	142	37	24
Mean No. $(C)/(B)$ of mf. $(C)/(A)$	79.1 11.11	67.5 8.40	62.1 6.79	33.1 3.26	27.1 2.14	28.7 1.73	20.1 0.82	15.8 0.32	7.4 0.08	12.0 0.06

and 1970 are compared in relation to microfilarial positives and negatives. The population in 1961 was 577 including 81 positives, while in 1970 it was 430 including 2 positives. Among the 81 positives in 1961, 49 turned to negative, 26 emigrated from the village and 5 died. One negative person turned to positive from 1964. Thus, there were only 2 positives in 1970. Because the population changed, the results of examinations on only the 266 persons who could be examined throughout the ten years from 1961 to 1970 are given in Tabled 4, which shows nearly the same trend in the reduction of microfilarial prevalence and density as that for all persons indicated in Table 2.

From the above, it can be said that in the Nagasaki area the eradication of bancroftian filariasis is possible by complete control of vec-

Table 3. Comparison of the Populations of Nagate Village between 1961 and 1970, in Relation to Microfilarial Positives and Negatives.

		Population in 1970			Emigrated (3)	Died (4)	(1)+(2)+(3)+(4)
		Mf (+) (1)	Mf (−) (2)	(1)+(2)			
Population in 1961	Mf (+) (1)	1	49	50	26	5	81
	Mf (−) (2)	1	284	285	181	30	496
	(1)+(2)	2	333	335	207	35	577
Immigrated (3)		0	46	46			
Born (4)		0	49	49			
(1)+(2)+(3)+(4)		2	428	430			

Table 4. Reduction of the Microfilarial Prevalence and Density in 60 mm³ Blood in 266 Persons Who Could be Examined throughout the Ten Years from 1961 to 1970 in Nagate Village.

Year	1961	1962	1963	1964	1965	1966	1967	1968	1969	1970
No. of mf. positives (A)	41	33	31	29	22	20	14	6	4	2
% mf. positives (A)/266 × 100	15.4	12.4	11.7	10.9	8.3	7.5	5.3	2.3	1.5	0.8
Total No. of mf. (B)	2,399	1,234	1,222	704	295	305	202	82	29	24
Mean No. (B)/(A)	58.5	37.4	39.4	24.3	13.4	15.3	14.4	13.7	7.3	12.0
of mf. (B)/266	9.02	4.64	4.59	2.65	1.11	1.15	0.76	0.31	0.11	0.09

tor mosquitoes, without treatment of persons with drugs. It is interesting that the eradication of the disease solely by controlling the
vector mosquitoes appears to require about nine years.

DECREASE IN EPIDEMIOLOGICAL DANGER
OF FILARIASIS INFECTION

The transmissibility of bancroftian filariasis by vector mosquitoes,
or the epidemiological danger of filariasis infection due to mosquitoes
to persons in a community, can be considered the product of three
factors: (1) effective microfilarial prevalence corrected in accordance with the microfilarial density in each person; (2) effective
period of transmission, and (3) abundance of vector mosquitoes
during the effective period (Omori and Wada, 1968). Here, the
effective microfilarial prevalence is obtained by dividing the total of
infection indices (anticipated infection rates of mosquitoes when fed
on each person in the village) by the total number of villagers.
The effective period of transmission is obtained by subtracting the
suppressed period for transmission of two months by residual spraying
of insecticide from the possible transmission period of three months
from late June to mid-September (Omori et al., 1967). Finally, the
abundance of vector mosquitoes during the effective period is obtained by finding the mean number of C. p. pallens females per house.

Table 5.　Yearly Changes in Epidemiological Danger of Filariasis
Infection in Persons in Nagate Village
(see text for epidemiological danger)

Year	Microfilarial prevalence (%)	Effective microfilarial prevalence (%) (1)	Effective months of transmission (2)	Mean no. of C. p. pallens per house (3)	Epidemi- ological danger (1) × (2) × (3)
1961	14.0	9.2	3.0	11.1	306.4
1962	12.4	7.7	1.4	1.5	16.2
1963	10.9	7.4	1.2	1.0	8.9
1964	9.8	5.5	1.1	0.2	1.2
1965	7.9	3.9	1.0	0.0	0.0
1966	6.0	3.5	1.3	0.1	0.5
1967	4.1	1.9	1.0	0.0	0.0
1968	2.0	0.9	1.0	0.4	0.4
1969	1.1	0.4	1.0	0.2	0.1
1970	0.5	0.2	1.0	0.0	0.0

In Table 5 is shown the yearly change in the epidemiological danger thus obtained. The effective microfilarial prevalence gradually decreased from 9.2 % in 1961 to 0.2 % in 1970. The effective period in months was 3.0 in 1961, and from 1.0 to 1.4 during and after 1962 because of residual spraying applied yearly in June (see Table 1). The mean number of $C. p. pallens$ females was as large as 11.1 in 1961, but was very small thereafter. The epidemiological danger of filariasis infection given by the product of the above three factors was as high as 306.4 in 1961, but decreased markedly to 16.2 in 1962, 8.9 in 1963, 1.2 in 1964, and nearly zero thereafter. This remarkable reduction in the epidemiological danger of filariasis infection is apparently mostly due to the notable decrease in the number of vector mosquitoes, and partly due to the gradual decrease in the effective microfilarial prevalance. Further, the greatly reduced epidemiological danger after 1962 would explain the gradual but steady reduction in microfilarial prevalence and density in persons of this village as shown in Tables 2 and 4, as filariasis infection would have occurred rarely, and adult filaria worms in humans would have died out gradually.

PERIOD DURING WHICH ADULT FILARIA WORMS CONTINUE TO PRODUCE MICROFILARIAE

During the experimental period of ten years from 1961 to 1970, there occurred great changes in the condition of the disease in each person. For example, some microfilarial positives turned to negative in the second year, some in the third year, and so on. Thus, the 266 persons who could be examined throughout the experimental period (see Table 4) are grouped on the basis of presence or absence of microfilariae every year from 1961 to 1970, and the yearly changes in the numbers, or mean numbers, of microfilariae in the respective groups are given in Table 6. All 37 persons from groups 1 to 10 were positive for microfilariae in 1961. Of these, 1 person from group 1 was continuously positive during the ten years, 1 person from group 2 turned to negative in 1970, 2 persons from group 3 in 1969, and so on. A total of 4 persons belonging to groups 11, 12, 13, and 14, though microfilariae were not found in 1962, 1964, 1963, and 1962, should perhaps be included in groups 4, 5, 7, and 8, respectively. Groups 15 to 21 each include one person negative in 1961 but becoming positive some years after by infection probably in 1961 or around that year

Table 6.　Yearly Changes in the Numbers or Mean Numbers of Microfilariae in 60 mm³ Blood by Group of 266 Persons Who Could Be Examined throughout the Ten Years from 1961 to 1970 in Nagate Village.

Group	1961	1962	1963	1964	1965	1966	1967	1968	1969	1970	No. of persons
1	20.0	16.0	55.0	42.0	34.0	37.0	52.0	53 0	15.0	23.0	1
2	171.0	68.0	49.0	61.0	13.0	25.0	4.0	4.0	1.0	0	1
3	32.0	20.0	11.5	12.5	17.5	14.0	5.0	1.5	0	0	2
4	68.8	53.3	55.7	43.5	18.7	16.3	8.0	0	0	0	6
5	39.8	38.0	78.0	31.0	12.0	6.0	0	0	0	0	4
6	38.7	36.0	50.7	10.7	2.5	0	0	0	0	0	3
7	189.4	68.0	32.8	16.8	0	0	0	0	0	0	5
8	107.0	14.7	9.3	0	0	0	0	0	0	0	3
9	17.2	5.2	0	0	0	0	0	0	0	0	5
10	7.0	0	0	0	0	0	0	0	0	0	7
11	16.0	0	11.0	10.0	16.0	19.0	9.0	0	0	0	1
12	30.0	60.0	38.0	0	1.0	7.0	0	0	0	0	1
13	1.0	2.0	0	1.0	0	0	0	0	0	0	1
14	6.0	0	5.0	0	0	0	0	0	0	0	1
15	0	58.0	26.0	9.0	0	0	0	0	0	0	1
16	0	0	23.0	46.0	20.0	31.0	2.0	0	0	0	1
17	0	0	0	3.0	8.0	28.0	75.0	20.0	11.0	1.0	1
18	0	0	0	4.0	0	5.0	2.0	2.0	2.0	0	1
19	0	0	2.0	0	0	0	0	0	0	0	1
20	0	0	0	2.0	0	3.0	0	0	0	0	1
21	0	0	0	0	1.0	0	0	0	0	0	1
22	0	0	0	0	0	0	0	0	0	0	218
No. of mf. positives	41	33	31	29	22	20	14	6	4	2	
% mf. positives	15.4	12.4	11.7	10.9	8.3	7.5	5.3	2.3	1.5	0.8	

within the village. A few persons may have been infected in neighboring villages with moderate filariasis endemicity (Wada, 1963). The 218 persons of group 22 were negative throughout the ten years.

The life span of adult filaria worms in humans is difficult to determine, but from Table 6 the mean period during which adults continue to produce microfilariae will be estimated as follows. In each of the seven years from 1962 to 1968, 7, 5, 3, 5, 3, 4, and 6 persons turned to negative in that order, but only 2 and 1 persons turned to negative in 1969 and 1970 respectively. This seems to indicate that the duration of time for continuous production of microfilariae by adult worms in humans is an average of approximately seven years.

In the case of the subperiodic *Wuchereria bancrofti* in the southern Pacific Islands, it was reported that 2–4 years is the average period during which a person remains positive for microfilariae as a result of a single infection (Hairston and Jachowsky, 1968; Hairston and Meillon, 1968), and microfilariae in persons persist less than 6 years after removal from the endemic area (Hu, 1952; Jachowsky *et al.*, 1951). These figures are fairly small compared with data on periodic *W. bancrofti* reported in the present paper, possibly because of the difference between periodic and subperiodic forms.

SUMMARY

The experiment in eradicating bancroftian filariasis was planned in 1962 to be carried out at Nagate Village solely through control of the vector mosquito, *Culex pipiens pallens*, and with no treatment of persons with drugs. From 1962 to 1970, residual spraying of insecticide of all dwellings and cowsheds was carried out once a year, and larvicide applications were repeated in all the breeding places of *C. p. pallens* in the village once a week every year during the breeding season of the vector mosquito. As a result of the control work, the density of the mosquito was suppressed to the level that new filaria infections were rarely found within the village. After 1961, all persons above one year of age were examined annually for microfilariae. In 1961 the number of villagers found positive for microfilariae was 81 out of 577, the positive rate having been 14.0%, the mean number of microfilariae for positives in 60 mm^3 blood was 79.1, and the average for all villagers 11.11. After 1962, when the vector mosquito control was started, microfilarial prevalence and density decreased gradually year by year, and in 1970 the positive rate was 0.5% and the mean numbers of microfilariae for positives and for all villagers were 12.0 and 0.06 respectively. Those results seem to be chiefly attributable to the natural death of adult filaria worms in carriers. From the above, it can be said that the eradication of bancroftian filariasis solely through control of vector mosquitoes is possible in about nine years. The period during which microfilariae can remain positive in respective carriers in the nearly complete absence of vector mosquitoes, is the duration of time for continuous production of microfilariae by adult worms in people. This period was estimated at an average of approximate seven years.

REFERENCES

Hairston, N. G. and Jachowski, L. A. (1968).   Analysis of the *Wuchereria bancrofti* population in the people of American Samoa. *Bull. Wld Hlth Org.*, **38**, 29.

Hairston, N. G. and Meillon, B. de (1968).   On the inefficiency of transmission of *Wuchereria bancrofti* from mosquito to human host. *Bull. Wld Hlth Org.*, **38**, 935.

Hu, S. M. K. (1952).   Mosquito control in the South Pacific. *Mosquito News*, **12**, 164.

Jachowski, L. A., Otto, G. F. and Wharton, J. D. (1951).   Filariasis in American Samoa. I. Loss of microfilaria in the absence of continued reinfection. *Proc. Helminthol. Soc.*, **18**, 25.

Omori, N. (1962).   A review of the role of mosquitos in the transmission of Malayan and Bancroftian filariasis in Japan. *Bull. Wld Hlth Org.*, **27**, 585.

Omori, N., Wada, Y., Oda, T. and Nishigaki, J. (1967).   Effects of experimental control work against vector mosquitoes of bancroftian filariasis in Japan. *Trop. Med.* (Nagasaki), **9**, 97.

Omori, N. and Wada, Y. (1968).   Factors affecting the transmissibility of bancroftian filariasis by mosquitoes. *Trop. Med.* (Nagasaki), **10**, 154.

Wada, Y. (1966).   Epidemiology of bancroftian filariasis in Nagate and Abumize Villages, Nagasaki Prefecture, especially in relation to vector mosquitoes. 2. Endemicity of the filariasis. *Endem. Dis. Bull. Nagasaki*, **5**, 136.

Wada, Y. (1966a).   Epidemiology of bancroftian filariasis in Nagate and Abumize Villages, Nagasaki Prefecture, especially in relation to vector mosquitoes. 3. Ecology and natural infection of mosquitoes. *Endem. Dis. Bull. Nagasaki*, **8**, 45.

Wada, Y. (1966b).   Epidemiology of bancroftian filariasis in Nagate and Abumize Villages, Nagasaki Prefecture, especially in relation to vector mosquitoes. 4. Filariasis eradication experiment by the control of vector mosquitoes. *Endem. Dis. Bull. Nagasaki*, **8**, 54.

Mass Treatment of Filariasis with Diethylcarbamazine in Endemic Areas in Kagoshima Prefecture

H. Sato, Y. Otsuji, T. Maeda, A. Nakashima and P. K. Yang

Second Department of Internal Medicine, School of Medicine,
Kagoshima University, Kagoshima, Japan

INTRODUCTION

In 1947 Hewitt *et al.* found 1-diethylcarbamyl-4-methyl-piperazine hydrochloride (Hetrazan), a piperazine derivative, to be effective for the eradication of microfilariae of some human filaria species such as *Wuchereria bancrofti* and *Brugia malayi*. Its effectiveness was later confirmed by other researchers. In Japan, Suganuma synthesized 1-diethylcarbamyl-4-methylpiperazine citrate (Supatonin) in 1951 and the drug has been proved by several workers to be very effective for the control of filariasis (Table 1).

Table 1.

1) Structure of Diethylcarbamazine (piperazine derivative)

1-diethylcarbamyl-4-methyl piperazine citrate

2) Structure of Hetrazon

1-diethylcarbamyl-4-methyl piperazine hydrochloride

Particular mention must be made of the advent of the drug, as it made mass treatment on microfilaria positive persons possible. We performed mass treatment of filarial patients with diethylcarbamazine in both Kiyohara and Shioya districts, Bonotsu, Kagoshima

[31]

Prefecture, putting special emphasis on careful and appropriate supervision of the drug administration. Districts where we performed mass treatment of microfilaria carriers were Kiyohara and Shioya in Bonotsu, Kagoshima prefecture, which lies in the southernmost part of Japan.

RESULTS

1. *Filarial surveys in Kiyohara district, Bonotsu*

The change in the microfilaria positive rate from 1954 through 1962 in Kiyohara district, which consists of the four villages of Sono, Kayano, Tatarazako and Hirahara, are shown in Table 2. In 1954 there were 60 microfilaria carriers out of 306 persons examined (microfilaria positive rate 19.6%) at Sono, 70 microfilaria carriers out of 441 persons examined (mf. positive rate 15.9%) at Kayano, 14 microfilaria carriers out of 236 persons examined (microfilaria positive rate 5.4%) at Tatarazako and 36 microfilaria carriers out of 452 persons examined (mf. positive rate 8.0%) at Hirahara.

To sum up, there were 180 microfilaria carriers out of 1435 persons examined (mf. positive rate 12.5%) in Kiyohara district. In 1959 the microfilaria positive rate at Sono was 16.4% (48 microfilaria carriers were found among 292 persons examined), 6.0% at Tatarazako (14 mf carriers out of 232 examined), 14.1% at Kayano (58 mf. carriers out of 412 persons examined) and 4.0% at Hirahara (17 mf. carriers out of 428 persons examined). The microfilaria positive rate in Kiyohara district in 1959 was therefore 10% (137 mf. carriers out of 1364 persons examined). The Japanese government, in 1962, decided to push an antifilarial campaign as a national policy. The microfilaria positive rate in 1962 in Kiyohara district was 8.6% (84 microfilaria carriers out of 972 persons examined). The breakdown was: 16.0% at Sono (36 microfilaria carriers out of 225 people examined), 10.0% at Kayano (32 microfilaria carriers out of 319 persons examined), 3.5% at Takarazako (5 microfilaria carriers out of 146 persons examined) and 3.9% at Hirahara (11 microfilaria carriers out of 283 people examined). The figures indicate that microfilaria positive rates were high at that time, though there was a tendency to decrease each year.

2. *Experimental mass treatment in both Kiyohara and Shioya districts, Bonotsu, Kagoshima prefecture*

Table 2. Results of Filarial Surveys Conducted in Kiyohara District Bonotsu, Kagoshima Prefecture, Japan

Year Village	1954			1959			1962		
	No. of persons examined	No. of Mf carriers	Mf positive rate	No. of persons examined	No. of Mf carriers	Mf positive rate	No. of persons examined	No. of Mf carriers	Mf positive rate
Sono	306	60	19.6%	292	48	16.4%	225	36	16.0%
Kayano	441	70	15.9	412	58	14.1	319	32	10.0
Tatarazako	236	14	5.4	232	14	6.0	145	5	3.5
Hirahara	452	36	8.0	428	17	4.0	283	11	3.9
Total	1435	180	12.5%	1364	137	10.0%	972	84	8.6%

Table 3.   Change in Mf Positive Rates in

Year \ Village	1962			MASS TREATMENT	1965	
	No. of persons examined	No. of Mf carriers	Mf positive rate		No. of persons examined	No. of Mf carriers
Sono	225	36	16.0%		222	9
Kayano	319	32	10.0		329	5
Tatarazako	145	5	3.5		197	3
Hirahara	283	11	3.9		316	1
Total	972	84	8.6%		1064	18

Table 4.   Change in Mf Positive rates in Kiyohara District, Bonotsu, Kagoshima Prefecture, Japan

Year	1962	1965	1967	1970
No. of persons examined	972	1064	922	802
No. of Mf carriers	84	18	4	0
Mf positive rate	8.6%	1.7	0.4	0
Total Mf count	2756	145	33	0
Average Mf count per capita	32.8	8.1	8.3	0
Mf residual rate	100%	5.3	1.2	0

Time of blood examination : 21.00–24.00

Blood quantity to be drawn from an earlobe for the examination : 30 mm^3 per capita

The method of the drug (diethylcarbamazine) administration was : 6mg/kg/day was administered as an initial dose for six consecutive days, followed by 6mg/kg/day, to be given once a week for six weeks amounting to 72mg/kg in total.

a. The experimental mass treatment conducted in Kiyohara district:

Results of investigations in 1962 conducted in Kiyohara district,

Kiyohara District, Bonotsu, Kagoshima Prefecture, Japan

	1967			1970		
Mf positive rate	No. of persons examined	No. of Mf carriers	Mf positive rate	No. of Persons examined	No. of Mf carriers	Mf positive rate
4.1%	201	1	0.5%	168	0	0
1.5	288	3	1.0	219	0	0
1.5	170	0	0	159	0	0
0.3	263	0	0	256	0	0
1.7%	922	4	0.4%	802	0	0

which consists of the four villages of Sono, Kayano, Tatarazako and Hirahara, in connection with filariasis show that the microfilaria positive rate was 8.6% in 1962 (84 microfilaria carriers were found out of 972 persons examined). The microfilaria carriers had been treated with 72mg/kg of diethylcarbamazine (Supatonin) in 1962. Three years later, in 1965, microfilaria positive rates in the district were proven to have decreased, as shown in Tables 3 and 4, and Fig. 1, to 4.1% at Sono (9 microfilaria carriers out of 222 persons examined), 1.5% at Kayano (5 microfilaria carriers out of 329 persons examined), 1.5% at Tatarazako (3 microfilaria carriers out of 197 persons examined) and 0.3% at Hirahara (only one microfilaria

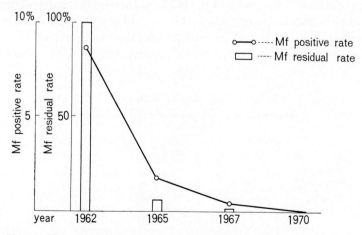

Fig. 1.   Change in Mf. Positive Rates and Mf. Residual Rates After Treatment in Kiyohara District.

carrier against 316 persons examined). The microfilaria positive rate in 1965 in Kiyohara district was reduced to 1.7% (18 microfilaria carriers against 1064 persons examined) from 8.6% on 1962 as a result of mass treatment with 72mg/kg of diethylcarbamazine (Supatonin). Later in 1967 only one microfilaria carrier out of 201 persons examined at Sono(microfilaria positive rate 0.5%) and 3 microfilaria carriers out of 288 persons examined at Kayano (microfilaria positive rate 1.0%) were found, though none of the microfilaria carriers were detected at either Tatarazake (170 persons examined) and Hirahara (263 persons examined). Collectively, the microfilaria positive rate in Kiyohara district in 1967 was 0.4% (4 microfilaria carriers out of 922 persons examined).

In 1970, 8 years after the first mass treatment with diethylcarbamazine in 1962, microfilaria carriers were not seen among examined people in all four villages (168 persons from Sono, 219 persons from Kayano, 159 persons from Tatarazako and 259 persons from Hira hara were examined).

b. The experimental mass treatment in Shioya district:

The microfilaria positive rate in Shioya district, Bonotsu, in 1958, as shown in Table 5, was found to be 13.3% as a result of investigtions (51 microfilaria carriers were detected out of 384 persons examined). As shown in Fig. 2, the 51 microfilaria carriers had been treated with 5mg/kg of diethylcarbamazine once a week for 10 weeks, and the microfilaria positive rate in 1959 was known to have been reduced to 5.4%, with 14 microfilaria carriers being detected out of 258 persons examined. These 14 microfilaria carriers were later administered 6mg/kg of diethylcarbamazine once a week for 5 weeks. As a result, the microfilaria positive rate in 1960 showed a

Table 5.   Change in Mf Positive Rates in Shioya District,
Bonotsu, Kagoshima Prefecture, Japan

Year	1958	1959	1960	1962	1965	1968
No. of persons examined	384	258	340	289	326	258
No. of Mf carriers	51	14	3	2	0	0
Mf positive rate	13.3%	5.4	0.9	0.7	0	0

remarkable decrease compared with that in 1959 (3 microfilaria carriers were detected out of 340 persons examined the microfilaria positive rate being 0.9%). The microfilaria positive rate in 1962 was 0.7% (2 microfilaria carriers out of 289 persons examined), though no microfilaria carriers were detected in 1965 (326 persons were examined) and in 1968 (258 persons were examined).

We now believe, based on the experimental mass treatment conducted by us in both Kiyohara and Shioya districts, Bonotsu, Kagoshima prefecture, Japan, that filariasis can be eradicated completely, provided the drug (diethylcarbamazine) administration procedure is conducted under careful and appropriate supervision of medical staff.

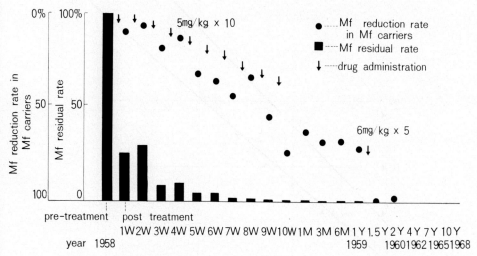

Fig. 2. Change in Mf. Reduction Rates and Mf. Residual Rates after Treatment in Shioya District. (1958–1968).

3. *Comparison of cumulative frequency distribution of microfilaria density in microfilaria carriers by pre-treatment and post-treatment surveys*

We will evaluate here the effect of diethylcarbamazine, based on the cumulative frequency distribution of microfilaria density in microfilaria carriers as presented by Sasa *et al.* (1964) and Kanda *et al.* (1966). Comparing cumulative frequency distribution of microfilaria density in microfilaria carriers in Kiyohara district, Bonotsu, in 1962 and that in 1965, higher cumulative frequency distribution is seen on the lower line showing low microfilaria density in Fig. 3 (horizontal

coordinate—logarithm of microfilaria density; vertical coordinate—
probit in %). On the other hand, the cumulative frequency distribution of microfilaria density in microfilaria carriers in Shioya district,
where the microfilaria positive rate was 13.3%, is higher on the line
showing low microfilaria density in Fig. 4 after administration of
25mg/kg of diethylcarbamazine than that before treatment. The
tendency is more marked after administration of 50mg/kg of diethylcarbamazine, which drug has been proven to be greatly effective for
the control of the disease in Japan.

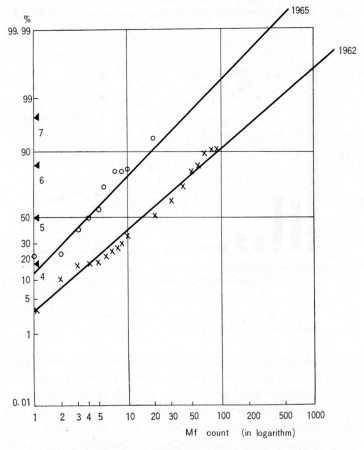

Fig. 3.   Cumulative Frequency Distribution of Mf. Density in Mf. Carriers in
Kiyohara District in 1962 and 1965.

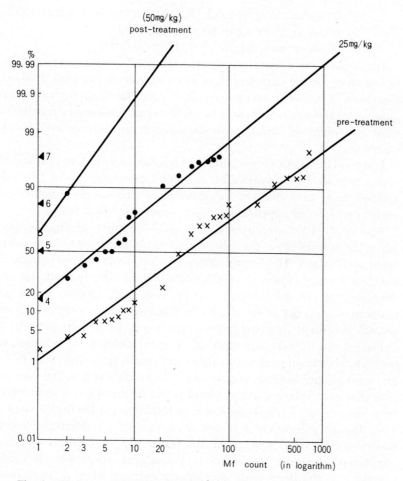

Fig. 4. Change in Cumulative Frequency Distribution of Mf. Density in Mf. Carriers after Treatment in Shioya District.

DISCUSSION

Remarkable results in the field of mass treatment of filarial patients have been obtained since Hewitt *et al.* first reported the effect of diethylcarbamazine. There have been several plans for mass treatment with diethylcarbamazine presented by researchers. They are:

1) 0.5–2.0mg/kg/day, taken on three occasions, for 2 or 3 weeks (Santiago-Stevenson, 1947).

    2) 0.3g/day, 5.0g in total (Kitamura and Katamine, 1952).
    3) 60mg or more/kg in total (Sasa, 1952).
    4) 70mg or more/kg in total (H. Sato, 1952).

Each plan mentioned above was reported by the researcher to be effective for the elimination of microfilariae in peripheral blood. Currently it has been recognized that 72mg/kg of diethylcarbamazine, in total dose, is sufficient to bring about satisfactory results for mass treatment of filarial patients without any serious side effects except fever.

It should be worth mentioning that microfilariae can be eradicated completely in 2 or 3 years after the first administration of Diethylcarbamazine, provided the administration procedure is conducted under careful and appropriate supervision of medical staff.

Sasa *et al.* (1959) reported that a small quantity of 2mg/kg/day, 30mg/kg in total dose, was also considerably effective for the treatment of filariasis. He further reported that, from the viewpoint of continued effectiveness of diethylcarbamazine, the microfilaria redeuction rate in microfilaria carriers was more striking when an equivalent quantity of the drug was administered intermittently for several months than when given continuously for a short period.

Fukushima (1963) investigated several schemes in relation to diethylcarbamazine administration and quantity of the drug to be given for proper mass treatment of filariasis. He came to the conclusion that microfilariae in the blood could be eliminated completely by administering 71mg/kg or more, in total dose, of Diethylcarbamazine, though effectiveness of the drug showed no difference when diethylcarbamazine was given intermittently or continuously, or combined. However, according to Fukushima, there were less side reactions to the drug with microfilaria carriers when a small dose (1.0–2.0mg/kg) of diethylcarbamazine was given as an initial dose, and increased gradually. In reality, however, it is continuous administration of diethylcarbamazine that is so often subject to neglect by filarial patients.

SUMMARY

It has been found that in both Kiyohara and Shioya districts, Bonotsu, Kagoshima prefecture, Japan, where 72mg/kg or more of diethylcarbamazine was administered to microfilaria carriers under careful and appropriate supervision of medical staff for the purpose of mass treatment of filarial patients, filariasis was almost completely controlled by the procedure of diethylcarbamazine administration alone.

REFERENCES

Edeson, J. F. B. and Wharton, R. H. (1958). Studies on filariasis in Malaya. Treatment of *Wuchereria malayi*-carriers with monthly or weekly doses of diethylcarbamazine (Banocide). *Ann. Trop. Med. & Parasit.*, **52**, 87.

Fukushima, H. (1963). Treatment of bancroftian filariasis with special emphasis on mass treatment. Proceedings of THE 16th GENERAL ASSEMBLY of THE JAPAN MEDICAL CONGRESS, Vol. 2, page 803.

Fukushima, H. and Yonamine, K. (1965). Studies on the Filariasis, 1. On the regional eradication of Bancroftian filariasis. Med. J. Kagoshima Univ. **17**, 3.

Hewitt, R. I., Kenng, M Chan, A. and Mohamed, A. (1950). Follow-up observations on the treatment of Bancroftian Filariasis with Hetrazan in British Guiana, *Am. J. Trop. Med.*, **30**, 217.

Hewitt, R. I., White, E., Wallage, W. S , Stewart, H. W., Kushner, S., and Subbarow, Y. (1947). Experimental Chemotherapy of filariasis, II Effect of piperazine derivative against naturally acquired filarial infection in cotton rats and dogs. *J. Lab. & Clin. Med.*, **32**, 1304.

Kanda, T. and Ishii, A. (1966). Evaluation of effects of deithylcabamazine administration to microfilaria positive cases in the control of Bancroftian filariasis in southern Amami Islands, Proc. Japan Soc. Trop. Med. **7**, 2.

Kenny, M. and Hewitt, R. I. (1949). Treatment of Bancroftian Filariasis with Hetrazane in British Guiana. *Am. J. Trop. Med.*, **29**, 89.

Otsuji, Y. (1954). A study of filariasis Report II. A study on wuchereriasis in the village of Bonotsu, Kagoshima Prefecture, Med. J. Kagoshima Univ.

Otsuji, Y. (1958). Experimental and Clinical studies on Wuchereriasis Bancrofti (Part II) Studies on filarial fever. Med. J. Kagoshima Univ., **10**, 4.

Santiago-Stevenson, D., Oliver-Gonzailz, J. and Hewitt, R. I. (1947). Treatment of filariasis bancrofti with I-diethylcarbamazine 1-4-methylpiperazine hydrochloride (Hetrazane). *J.A.M.A.*, **135**, 708.

Sasa, M., Sato, K., Osada, Y., Ikeshoji, T., Fukushima, H., Yonezawa, T., Tanaka, H., Hori, E., Komine, I., Izumi, K. and Iwai, K. (1959). Studies on the control of bancroftian filariasis in Amami Oshima island. *Jap. J. Parasit.*, Vol. 8, No. 6.

Sasa, M. and Mitsui, G. (1964). Frequency distribution of the microfilaria densities of people in the endemic areas of bancroftian filariasis in the Amami Islands, south Japan. *Jap. J. Exp. Med.*, **34**, 17.

Sato, H. (1965). Review on the Therapy of Filariasis. *Acta Med. Univ. Kagoshima*, **7**, 173.

Sato, H. and Otsuji, Y. (1954). Filariasis. *Internal Medicine*, **16**, 70.

Sato, H. and Yonezawa, T. (1954). Filariasis. *Japan. J. Clin. and Exp. Med.*, **31**, 5.

Sato, H., Yonezawa, T., Fukushima, H., Otsuji, Y. and Kijima, T. (1958). A Study on filariasis (Report 21) Results 5 years after the mass therapy by Supatonin. Med. J. Kagoshima Univ. Vol. 9, No. 6.

Yamamoto, H. (1965). Studies on epidemiology of filariasis III. Comparative studies of the effect of diethylcarbamazine on the microfilarial carriers administered at different doses and intervals. Japan. J. Parasit. Vol. 14, No. 2.

Yonamine, K. (1964). Studies on mass treatment of filariasis. Med. J. Kagoshima Univ., Vol. 16, No. 1.

The Ultrastructure of Mosquitoes
4. Flight muscle of *Culex pipiens pallens*

Y. Tongu, S. Suguri, D. Sakumoto, K. Itano
and S. Inatomi

Department of Parasitology, Okayama University Medical School, Japan

INTRODUCTION

The ultrastructural features of insect flight muscles have been described in a number of previous publications [for example, Chapman (1954) for firefly, fruitfly, housefly, wasp; Philpott and Szentgyörgyi (1955) for housefly, bumble bee; Smith (1963, 1965, 1966) for blowfly, aphid, *Odonata*; Simon *et al.* (1969) for housefly]. Among them Simon *et al.* showed the characteristic changes of mitochondria in flight muscles.

In recent years, mosquitoes have been studied morphologically by Bertram and Bird (1961), Clements and Potter (1967); Tongu *et al.* (1968, 1969), and Suguri *et al.* (1969), but there have been no reports on mosquito flight muscles. Although ultrastructural features of the larvae of *Brugia pahangi* in mosquito flight muscles were described by Beckett and Boothroyd (1970), and they suggested that the mitochondria of the flight muscles were eaten by the larvae of *B. pahangi*, the characteristic pattern of the flight muscle has not been established beyond that of the mitochondria.

The present paper lays the groundwork for tracing the relationship between mosquito and microfilariae.

MATERIALS AND METHODS

The mosquitoes (*Culex pipiens pallens* Coquillet, 1898) were taken from a colony of OK701 that are the offspring of many inbred generations of a standard laboratory strain originally supplied by the Parasitology Laboratory of Okayama University. Adult mosquitoes were maintained on sugar and water at 27°C. Before dissection the mosquitoes were kept in an ice box for a few minutes to be anesthetized. Flight muscles dissected from the thorax were fixed for 2 hours

[43]

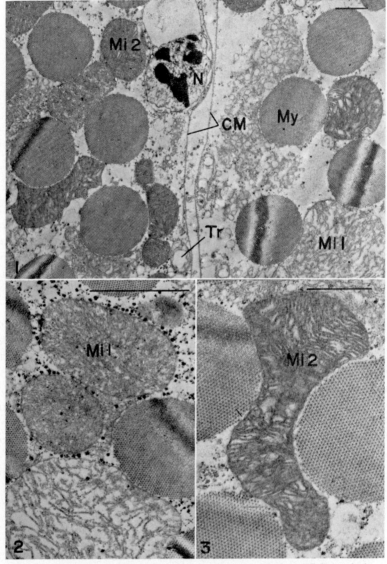

Fig. 1.   Cross-Section of the Muscle Fiber. Showing a Nucleus (N) Beneath the
Cell Membrane (CM), Two Types of Mitochondria (Mi1, Mi2), the Tracheas
(Tr), and Many Myofibrils (My).
There can be seen the swellings and fenestrations of mitochondria.
Fig. 2.   Type 1 Mitochondria (Mi) with Simple Cristae and Light Matrix
Surrounded by Many Glycogen Granules.
Fig. 3.   Type 2 Mitochondrion (Mi2) with Complex Cristae and Dense Matrix.
                                    (Scale is 1 micron in the micrograph)

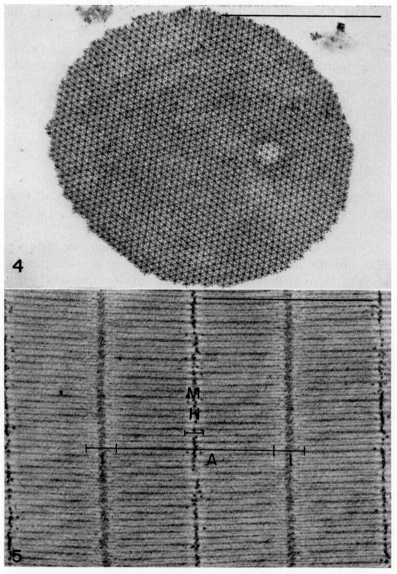

Fig. 4. Cross-Section of a Myofibril.
Showing the regular pattern of thick and thin myofilaments.
Fig. 5. Longitudinal Section of a Myofibril.
There can be seen A, I, H, and M bands.

(Scale is 1 micron in the micrograph)

with 1.25% cold glutaraldehyde in phosphate buffer (pH 7.4). The tissues were then rinsed with the same buffer and postfixed for 1 to 2 hours with 2% osmium tetroxide in phosphate buffer (pH 7.4). They were dehydrated in increasing concentrations of ethanol in water and finally placed in propylene oxide. They were embedded in Epon. Thin sections were cut on a Porter-Blum Ultramicrotome and stained with lead nitrate and uranyl acetate. They were examined with a Hitachi HS-8 electron microscope.

RESULTS

The flight muscle cell has a thin cell membrane (Fig. 1, CM) about 300 Å in thickness. It is not certain whether the membrane has a double or a single structure.

The nerve endings and the trachea (Fig. 1, Tr) are located on the cell membrane, and the axons are sometimes found in close association with the muscle fiber. The trachea with conspicuous taenidia passes through single or groups of muscle fibers.

The muscle cell consists of a great mass of parallel myofibrils, 1,000 to 3,000 in number and 2 μ in diameter. These myofibrils (Fig. 1, My) are loosely packed in the sarcoplasmic matrix, and large mitochondria with complex multicristae are arranged between the myofibrils.

A great majority of the nuclei (Fig. 1, N) of the cells lie just beneath the cell membrane. Occasionally, however, more centrally located nuclei are seen.

In all specimens two kinds of mitochondria are observed, but also some intermediate forms can be seen. Type 1 (Figs. 1, 2, Mi 1) has simply folded cristae and light matrix, and type 2 (Figs. 1, 3, Mi2), with the cristal structure surrounded by a dense matrix, has the cristal membrane folded and woven into an exceedingly complex pattern.

In some specimens the mitochondria show swelling due to an increase of intracristal spaces. Glycogen granules are seen in the sarcoplasmic matrix.

In cross-section (Fig. 4) at the level of the A band, the myofibrils are composed of a regular hexagonal array of thick and thin myofilaments.

The point-like profiles of six thin filaments are evenly spaced around each thick filament. The thicker filament is about 170 Å and the thinner about 70 Å in diameter. In longitudinal section (Fig. 5) of the muscle fibers the myofibrils show striated muscle as regular bands.

The dark bands are anisotropic (A bands) and therefore appear bright whereas the light bands are isotropic (I band) and appear dark. The A band has the H band in its center, and the M band is in the center of the H band. The A band is composed of thick and thin myofilaments. The H band consists of thick filaments, and the light I band bisected by the Z line is composed of thin myofilaments only.

DISCUSSION

During the course of the study of the flight muscles of insects, Smith (1965) and Simon *et al.* (1969) recorded that the mitochondria and myofibrils are loosely arranged together. In our observation mosquito flight muscle has been found to have the same arrangement, although the fibrils and mitochondria are more closely packed in dragonflies and damselflies (Smith, 1966).

Chapman (1954) observed the sarcolemma appearing as a thin limiting membrane. In mosquito flight muscle the unit membrane was observed to be the so-called sarcolemma.

The fine structure of the mitochondria in flight muscles was studied by Chapman (1954), Philpott and Szent-györgi (1955), Smith (1966), and Simon *et al.* (1969). Simon *et al.* reported that the mitochondria of the mosquito differ in shape and number according to age. Furthermore, they distinctly observed two kinds of mitochondria in *Musca domestica* L.. Type 1 has simple folded cristae and a light matrix. The whole area of type 2 cristal membrane is far greater than in type 1.

In the present paper, two types of mitochondria were recognized, but the intermediate form between the two types was also described for all specimens. The entire mitochondria, therefore, were not strictly classified into two groups.

Mitochondria of the wing muscle of the bumble-bee show a tubular inner structure, while the mitochondria of the leg muscle show laminar formations (Philpott and Szent-györgyi, 1955). In mosquito flight muscle, type 2 mitochondria clearly shows laminar cristae. Type 1 appears to be of tubular-like cristae.

In some specimens these mitochondria show swelling and fenestration. The mitochondria in flight muscles seem to degenerate by swelling and fenestration as in the case of housefly (Simon *et al.*, 1969).

SUMMARY

The mosquitoes were refrigerated for a few minutes and then fixed with 1.25% glutaraldehyde for 2 hours in the ice box. They were then postfixed with 2% osmium tetroxide for 2 hours. The tissues were dehydrated with ethanol series by routine methods and were embedded in Epon. Thin sections were stained with uranyl acetate and lead nitrate.

In the present paper the normal fine structure of the mosquito flight muscle is described. Myofibrils and mitochondria of flight muscles having a thin unit membrane are loosely arranged in the sarcoplasmic matrix. Muscle fibers having about 1,000 to 3,000 myofibrils show a regular band and a pattern similar to the striated muscle cell, namely the myofibril consisting of thick and thin myo-filaments has A, I, Z, M, and H bands. Two types of mitochondria with intermediate type were seen in the flight muscle: type 1 with simple tubular-like cristae and light matrix, and type 2 with complex laminar cristae and a dense matrix. Some mitochondria show fenest-rations among the cristal membranes and swelling.

REFERENCES

Beckett, E. S. and Boothroyd, B. (1970).   Mode of nutrition of the larvae of the filarial nematode *Brugia pahangi*. *Parasitology*, **60**, 21.

Bertram, D. S. and Bird R. G. (1961).   Studies on mosquito-borne viruses in their vectors. 1) The normal fine structure of the midgut epithelium of the adult female *Aedes aegypti*(L.) and the functional significance of its modification following a blood meal. *Trans. R. Soc. Trop. Med. Hyg.*, **55**, 404.

Chapman, G. B. (1954).   Electron microscopy of ultra-thin sections of insect flight mus-cle. *J. Morph.*, **95**, 237.

Clements, A. N. and Potter, S. A. (1967).   The fine structure of the spermathecae and their ducts in the mosquito *Aedes aegypti*. *J. Insect Physiol.*, **13**, 1825.

Philpott, D. E. and Szent-györgyi, A. (1955).   Observations on the electron microscopic structure of insect muscle. *Biochem. Biophys. Acta*, **18**, 177.

Simon, J., Bhatnagar, P. L. and Milburn, N. S. (1969).   An electron microscope study of changes in mitochondria of flight muscle of ageing houseflies (*Musca domestica*). *J. Insect Physiol.*, **15**, 135.

Smith, D. S. (1963).   The structure of flight muscle salcosomes in the blowfly *Calliphora erythrocephala* (Diptera). *J. Cell Biol.*, **19**, 115.

Smith, D. S. (1965).   Organization of flight muscle in an aphid, *Megoura viciae* (Homop-tera). *J. Cell Biol.*, **27**, 379.

Smith, D. S. (1966).   The organization of flight muscle fibers in the *Odonata*. *J. Cell Biol.*, **28**, 109.

Suguri, S., Tongu, Y., Sakumoto, D., Itano, K. and Inatomi, S. (1969). The ultrastructure of mosquitoes. 2. Malpighian tubule of *Culex pipiens pallens*. *Jap. J. Sanit.
Zool.*, **20**, 1.

Tongu, Y., Suguri, S., Sakumoto, D., Itano, K. and Inatomi, S. (1968). The ultrastructure of mosquitoes. 1. Spermatozoa in *Culex pipiens pallens*. *Jap. J. Sanit. Zool.*,
19, 215.

Tongu, Y., Suguri, S., Sakumoto D., Itano, K., and Inatomi, S. (1969). The ultrastructure of mosquitoes. 3. Hindgut of *Aedes aegypti*. *Jap. J. Sanit. Zool.*, **20**, 168.

The Ultrastructure of Mosquitoes
5. Salivary gland of *Culex tritaeniorhynchus*

S. Suguri, Y. Tongu, D. Sakumoto, K. Itano
and S. Inatomi

Department of Parasitology, Okayama University Medical School, Japan

INTRODUCTION

Mosquitoes serve as cyclic or mechanical vectors of important helminthic, protozoan, bacterial and viral diseases. Many parasitologists and biologists have been interested in the vector-host-parasite relationship. Concerning filariasis, there are many morphological, histochemical, and immunological studies on the development of larvae in the mosquito, and the changes of structure and function in mosquito tissues.

We have been studying this vector-host-parasite relationship with the electron microscope. First, we observed normal tissues of uninfected mosquitoes. Many reports on the normal structures of mosquitoes are available such as that on the mid-gut by Bertram *et al.* (1961), on the spermatheca by Clements and Potter (1967), on the spermatozoa by Tongu *et al.* (1968), on the malpighian tubule by Suguri *et al.* (1969), on the hind-gut by Tongu *et al.* (1969), and on the flight muscle by Tongu *et al.* (in press). In the present investigation, the salivary gland of *Culex tritaeniorhynchus* was studied.

MATERIALS AND METHODS

The materials used in this study were adult *C. tritaeniorhynchus* obtained from the mosquito colony of our department. In this colony, sugar water was given to adults, solid food usually given to rats was given to larvae, and as a source of blood meal, hamsters were used. Female adults (20–40 days after emergence, 10–30 days after engorging) were dissected in cold saline, and their salivary glands were rapidly transferred to an ice-cold solution of 1.25% glutaraldehyde in 0.1 M phosphate buffer (pH 7.4). Tissues were fixed in glutaraldehyde solution for 30 min. washed with the same phosphate buffer, and post-fixed for 2 hr. at 5°C with 1% osmium tetroxide in 0.1 M phosphate buffer (pH 7.6). After fixation, the tissues were dehydrated with a graded series of ethanols followed by propylene oxide and embedded in Epon. Polymerization occurred overnight at 60°C. Thin sections were cut with glass knives on a Porter-Blum microtome, and stained in saturated aqueous uranyl acetate, counterstained with lead nitrate. Sections were examined with a Hitachi HS-8 electron microscope.

RESULTS

1. *General morphology of the gland*

A pair of salivary glands lies in front of the thorax. Each gland is composed of three lobes, two lateral (about 420 μ in length) and one median (about 360 μ in length). All three lobes are clearly demarcated into anterior and posterior regions. Orr *et al.* (1961) called the anterior regions "necks" and the posterior regions, "acini". The median neck is about 5 μ in length and the lateral 17 μ.

The gland is covered with a basement membrane measuring about 900 Å in thickness. Each lobe consists of a single layer of cells placed around an intraglandular duct. This cuticular duct is about 2 μ in diameter and extends almost the full length of each of the lobes. Each duct is joined to the cuticular duct of the salivary duct and extends to the neck region of the mosquito.

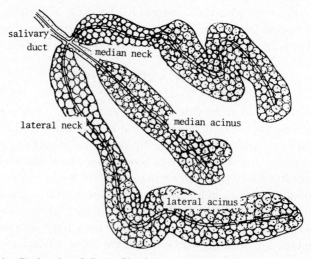

Fig. 1.   Regions in a Salivary Gland.

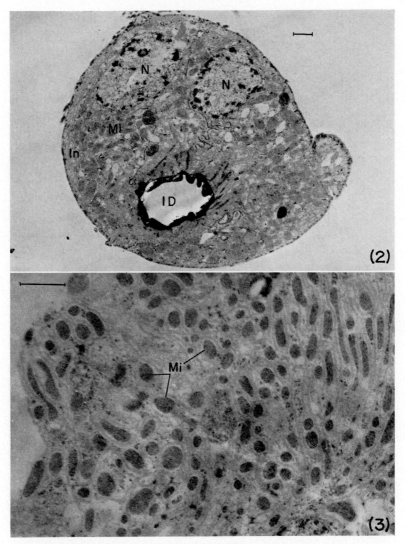

Fig. 2.   Transverse Section of Salivary Duct.

The duct is covered with a basement membrane. Infolding (In) of the cell membrane is frequent at the periphery of the duct. The cytoplasm among these infoldings is filled with many mitochondria (Mi). N: Nucleus, ID: Intraglandular Duct. Scale: 1μ.

Fig. 3.   Peripheral Portion of Salivary Duct.

The cell membrane infolds frequently and to a considerable extent, and among the infoldings many mitochondria (Mi) are present. Scale: 1μ.

54   S. SUGURI ET AL.

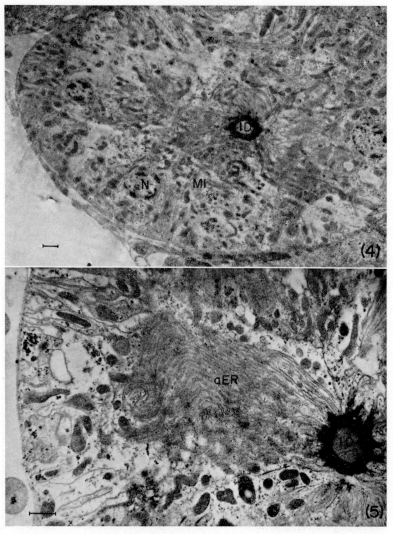

Fig. 4.   Transverse Section of Median Neck.
The infolding of cell membrane is seen, but it is not as frequent as in the salivary duct. Many mitochondria (Mi) are present. N: Nucleus, ID: Intraglandular Duct. Scale: 1μ.
Fig. 5.   A kind of agranular endoplasmic reticulum (aER) is connected to an
intraglandular duct wall (ID). Scale: 1μ.

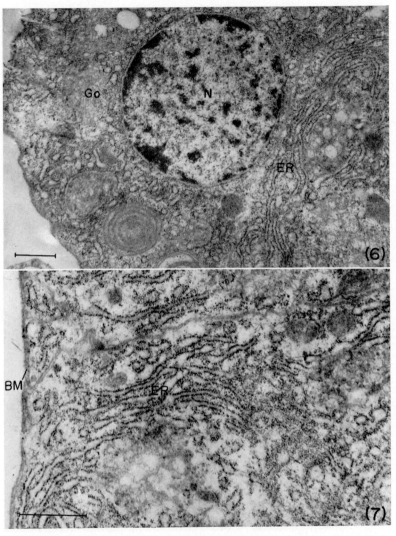

Fig. 6.   Transverse Section of the Antero-lateral Neck.
   Cytoplasm is filled with granular endoplasmic reticula (ER).
   Some Golgi complexes (Go) and vacuoles are scattered. N: Nucleus. Scale: 1μ.
Fig. 7.   Peripheral Region of the Antero-lateral Neck.
   Cytoplasm is full of granular endoplasmic reticula (ER). BM: Basement
Membrane. Scale: 1μ.

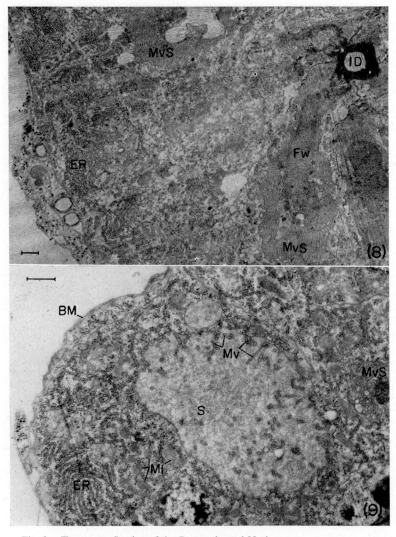

Fig. 8.   Transverse Section of the Postero-lateral Neck.

Granular endoplasmic reticula (ER) are present at the periphery of the acinus, and feltworks (Fw) connecting with an intraglandular duct (ID) extend into the gland cells, with microvilli systems (MvS) surrounding feltworks. The cuticular-duct wall has holes. Scale: 1μ.

Fig. 9.   Peripheral Region of Gland Cell in the Postero-lateral Neck.

Microvilli (Mv) can be seen extending into secretion. The cytoplasm around the secretion is filled with granular endoplasmic reticula (ER) and mitochondria (Mi). MvS: Microvilli system, BM: Basement membrane. Scale: 1μ.

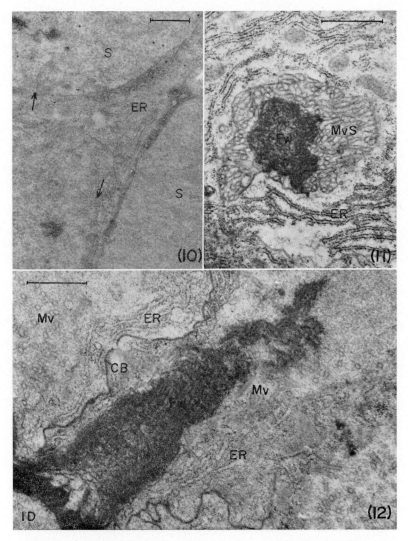

Fig. 10. A Part of the Secretion (S) Remote from the Intraglandular Duct.
Note some microvilli branching from one point. (arrow) ER: Granular Endoplasmic Reticulum. Scale: 1μ.

Fig. 11. Feltworks are surrounded by the microvilli system (MvS). In a part where secretion is not observed, the microvilli tightly surround the feltwork (Fw).

Fig. 12. Feltwork Extending into Secretion. The feltwork connects to an intraglandular duct wall, and the duct wall has a hole at the connecting point. The cell membrane having microvilli (Mv) surrounds the secretion. The cytoplasm forming a rim arround the secretion is filled with granular endoplasmic reticula (ER). ID: Intragrandular Duct, CB: Cell Boundary. Scale: 1μ.

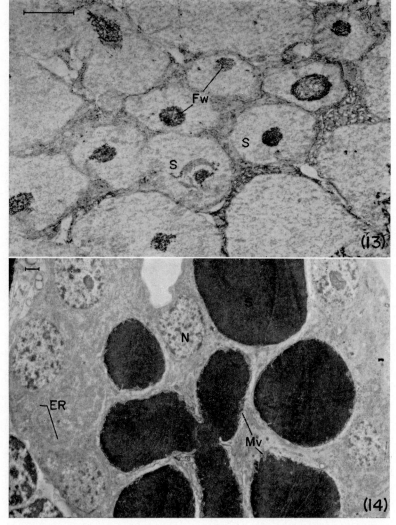

Fig. 13. Longitudinal Section at the Adjacent Part of the Intraglandular Duct in the Postero-Lateral Neck.

This photograph shows each feltwork (Fw) extending into each secretion (S). Scale: 1μ.

Fig. 14. Transverse Section of the Central Acinus Near the Neck.

Secretion is of high-electron density. Nuclei exist at the periphery of the gland, but cytoplasm filled with granular endoplasmic reticula (ER) forms considerable space. Microvilli (Mv) are present at the limb of the secretion. Scale: 1μ.

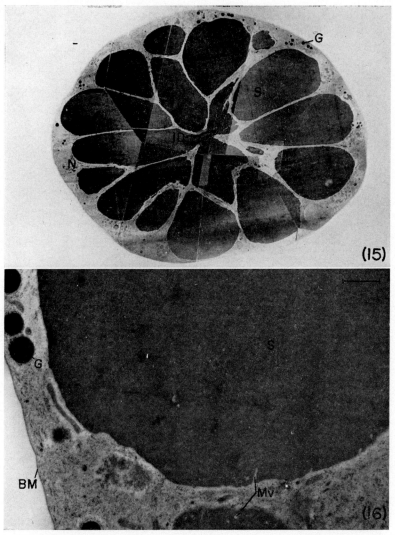

Fig. 15.　Transverse Section of Central Acinus.

Secretion occupies almost all the space of the section, and at the periphery of the acinus, nuclei and electron-dense granules (G) are observed. Scale: 1μ.

Fig. 16.　Peripheral Regions of Lateral Acinus.

Electron-dense granules (G) can be seen and around these granules many free ribosomes are scattered. A basement membrane (BM) is seen covering the acinus. Mv: Microvillus. Scale: 1μ.

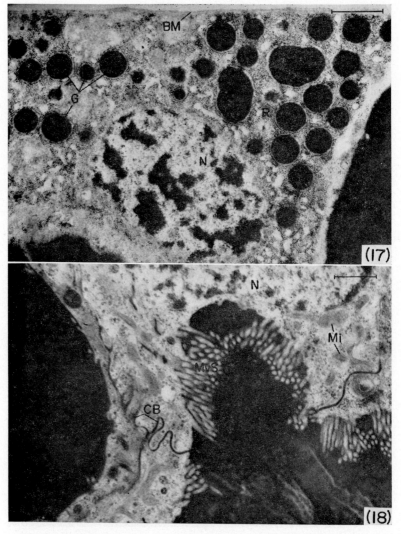

Fig. 17.   Peripheral Regions of Lateral Acinus.

Electron-dense granules (G) can be seen and around these granules many free ribosomes are scattered. A basement membrane (BM) is seen covering the acinus. N: Nucleus. Scale: 1μ.

Fig. 18.   Microvilli System in the Lateral Acinus.

The secretion is high-electron dense, so the border of the microvillus is not distinct. The cell boundary (CB) appears as an electron-dense line. N: Nucleus, Mi: Mitochondrion. Scale: 1μ.

In the transverse section of the salivary duct two or three cells are found, and the number of cells increases as the section approaches the end of the lobes. At the acini, about 20 cells are observed.

The gland may be divided into four regions; the salivary duct, median neck, lateral neck, and median and lateral acini.

2. The fine Structure of the salivary gland cells
a. Salivary duct

The salivary duct is about 15 μ in diameter and two or three epithelial cells are distributed around a cuticular duct measuring 2 μ in diameter, 0.5 μ in thickness in transverse section. The wall of the intraglandular duct has a simple structure of high electron density. These duct cells are underlaid with a basement membrane. The most striking feature of this cell is that the cell membrane is infolded at the peripheral part of the salivary duct. The cytoplasm in these infoldings is filled with numerous mitochondria, and the cell boundary is clearly apparent.

b. Median neck

The fine structure of the epithelial cells forming the median neck resembles closely that of the salivary duct cells just described. The basal surface of a lobe is covered with a basement membrane about 900 Å thick. The underlying basal cell membrane is considerably infolded into the cytoplasm. Mitochondria of various shapes, 0.5–2 μ in length, are found among the infoldings of the cell membrane. A kind of agranular endoplasmic reticulum in parallel array and of considerable length (up to about 12 μ) is found around the intraglandular duct. The outer surface of cuticle of the intraglandular duct is uneven, but the inner surface is simple. Borders of cells are clearly found.

c. Lateral neck

The lateral neck is divided into two regions; namely, anterior and posterior regions. The fine structure of the cell in the anterior region is similar to that in the salivary duct or the median neck. But the infolding of cell membrane is not as well developed as in the salivary duct or the median neck, and many granular endoplasmic reticula exist. The cytoplasm is filled with many granular endoplasmic reticula, mitochondria and vacuoles of various shapes. A few Golgi complexes are also found scattered sparsely. The shape of the cuticular wall of the intraglandular duct is not complicated. The primary difference between the posterior region and the anterior is that secretion exists in the posterior. The density of this secretion is low, and coagulated dot-like substances of high-electron density are scattered all around the secretion. Each cell is largely filled with secretion while its nucleus and the other organelles are displaced to the periphery of the gland and some cytoplasm is distributed as a scarcely-perceptible rim at the margin. The wall of the intraglandular duct has many holes (about 0.15 μ in diameter), and the outer surface of the wall is irregular. The wall is connected to feltworks extending considerably far into the secretion. It is composed of electron-dense fibrous materials (about 150 Å in diameter), and the density of the fibrous material is low at the tip of the feltwork. Each glandular cell has an inner region composed of a microvilli system underneath which secretion is stored. The secretion exists between the microvilli layer and the feltwork. When secretion exists, the innerside cell membrane extends into the cell itself, and the microvilli are sparse in this region. When secretion is not stored, the microvilli tightly surround the feltwork and the density of microvilli is high. The microvillus is 0.12 μ in diametre. The feltwork connects to the outer surface of the intraglandular duct wall, and between these structures a zone of low-electron density exists. The duct wall is electron-dense and the lumen content gives the same appearance as the secretion.

d. Median acinus and lateral acinus

The median acinus and the lateral acinus have cells of the same structure. Cells of these acini have secretion and granules of high-electron density. Except this feature, the fine structure of the cell is similar to that of the postero-lateral neck. Each cell is largely filled with secretion, and its nucleus, granular endoplasmic reticula and other cytoplasmic organelles are displaced to the periphery of the gland. Microvilli are found as in the postero-lateral neck, but the secretion is so electron-dense that the edge of microvillus and the feltwork are not as distinct. The secretion in the lumen is a homogeneous substance of high-electron density and the same as the adjacent secretion. Concerning electron-density, more than two kinds of secretion are observed. In the cytoplasm, electron-dense granules (0.2–2 μ in diameter) are found, and around these granules many free ribosomes are scattered.

DISCUSSION

Shishiliaeva-Matova (1942) reported that three distinct secretory regions are present in each gland of Culicinae: in the median acinus, the lateral acini, and the lateral necks. From histochemical tests on the salivary glands of *Aedes aegypti* females, Orr *et al.* (1961) concluded that the central acinus secretes a conjugated muccopolysaccharide, and the lateral acini a carbohydrate-protein complex as well as a protein. The nucleoli of the central and lateral acini become greatly enlarged and there is an increase in RNA around the nuclei 24 hours after taking a blood meal. Metcalf (1945) reported that digestive enzymes are not found in the salivary glands and division of the salivary gland shows that agglutinin of erythrocytes is produced only by the median lobe. The present study indicates that four principal structural regions exist in the mature salivary glands of the female mosquito: the salivary duct, the central and antero-lateral necks, the postero-lateral neck, and the lateral and median acini have secretion. In the lateral neck, the electron-density of the secretion is low, while in the lateral and median acini the electron-density is high, but the density varies somewhat. The difference between the median acinus secretion and the lateral is not clear.

Clements and Potter described the feltwork and microvilli in the spermathecae of female *Aedes aegypti*. According to their paper one end of each glandular cell is filled with a mass of microvilli, and converges on a ductule which holds feltwork. Secretion is not found near the microvilli or the feltwork, but in the lateral neck of the salivary gland. The secretion is stored between a microvilli system and a feltwork, and the feltwork (up to 20 μ) is longer and more electron-dense than in the case of a spermatheca.

Kloetzel and Laufer (1969) discussed the fine structure of the larval salivary gland in *Chironomus*. The gland has an apical brush border at the apical region, but does not have the feltwork and the cuticular duct.

SUMMARY

The salivary gland is covered with a basement membrane. Each lobe consists of a single layer of cells disposed around an intraglandular duct, and this cuticular duct extends almost the full length of each lobe.

The gland may be divided into four regions: the salivary duct, median neck, lateral neck, and median and lateral acini.

The salivary duct (about 15 μ in diameter) has two or three epithelial cells in a transverse section. At the basal part, the cell membrane is frequently infolded, and cytoplasm among these infoldings is filled with mitochondria.

The epithelial cells forming the median neck are similar to those in the salivary duct. But a kind of agranular endoplasmic reticulum is observed around the intraglandular duct.

The lateral neck is divided into two regions. The structure of the cell at the anterior region is similar to that of the salivary duct. But the infolding of cell membrane is not as well developed as in the salivary duct, and in the cytoplasm many granular endoplasmic reticula are observed. The cell in the posterior region has secretion of low electron density. Each cell is filled with the secretion while the organelles are displaced to the periphery of the gland and cytoplasm is distributed like a rim at the margin of the secretion. Each cell has a microvilli system at the inner region, and the microvilli are sparse at the region remote from the intraglandular duct. The wall of the intraglandular duct has many holes and it connects with feltworks composed of electron-dense fibrous substances. Secretion exists between the microvilli layer and the feltwork.

The structure of the median acinus is the same as that of lateral acinus. These acini have secretion and granules (0.2–2 μ in diameter) of high-electron density but the electron density of these secretions varies somewhat.

REFERENCES

Bertram, D. S. and Bird, R. G. (1961). Studied on mosquito-borne viruses in their vectors. I. The normal fine structure of the midgut epithelium of the adult female *Aedes aegypti* (L.) and the functional significance of its modification following a blood meal. *Trans. R. Soc. Trop. Med. Hyg.*, **55**, 404.

Bhatia, M. L., Wattal, B. L., and Kalra, N. L. (1957). Structure of salivary glands in mosquitoes. *Ind. J. Malar.*, **11**, 55.

Clements, A. N. (1963). The Physiology of Mosquitoes. Macmillan and Co., New York.

Clements, A. N. and Potter, S. A. (1967). The fine structure of the spermathecae and their ducts in the mosquito *Aedes aegypti*. *J. Insect Physiol.*, **13**, 1825.

Kloetzel, J. A. and Laufer, H. (1969). A fine-structural analysis of larval salivary gland function in *Chironomus thummi* (Diptera). *J. Ultrastruct. Res.*, **29**, 15.

Metcalf, R. L. (1945). The physiology of the salivary glands of *Anopheles quadrimaculatus*. *J. Nat. Marlar. Soc.*, **4**, 271.

Orr, C. W. M., Hudson, A., and West, A. S. (1961). The salivary glands of *Aedes aegypti*. Histological-histochemical studies. *Can. J. Zool.*, **39**, 265.

Phillips, M., David and Swift, Hewson (1965). Cytoplasmic fine structure of *Sciara* salivary glands. *J. Cell Biol.*, **27**, 395.

Schin, Ssu Ki and Clever, Ulrich (1967). Ultrastructural and cytochemical studies of salivary gland regression in *Chironomus tentans*. *Zeit. S. Zellforsch.*, **86**, 262.

Shishliaeva-Matova, Z. S. (1942). Comparative study of *Culicinae* salivary glands of the Samarkand District. Report I. Histology and comparative morphology mosquito salivary glands. *Med. Parasit., Moscow*, **11**, 61.

Suguri, S., Tongu, Y., Itano, K., Sakumoto, D., and Inatomi, S. (1969). The Ultra structure of mosquitoes. 2. Malpighian tubule of *Culex pipiens pallens*. *Jap. J. Sanit. Zool.*, **20**, 1.

Tongu, Y., Suguri, S., Itano, K., Sakumoto, D., and Inatomi, S. (1968). The Ultra-structure of mosquitoes. 1. Spermatozoa in *Culex pipiens pallens*. *Jap. J. Sanit. Zool.*, **19**, 215.

Tongu, Y., Suguri, S., Sakumoto, D., Itano, K., and Iantomi, S. (1969). The Ultra-structure of mosquitoes. 3. Hindgut of *Aedes aegypti*. *Jap. J. Sanit. Zool.*, **20**, 168.

Observations on Some American Poeciliid Fish Established in Polluted Waters in Japan and South Asia, with Special Reference to Their Use in the Control of Filaria Vectors*

M. SASA

*Department of Parasitology, the Institute of Medical Science,
University of Tokyo, Tokyo, Japan*

INTRODUCTION

It has been known for many years that some fresh water fish are an efficient natural enemy of mosquito larvae and can be used as a means of biological control of some mosquito-borne diseases. A comprehensive review was made by Gerberich and Laird (1966) on the control of mosquitoes by the use of fish. Among these, the most familiar is the introduction of the top minnow, *Gambusia affinis* (Baird et Girard, 1853), into many countries in Europe, Africa and Asia from its native southern United States, for the purpose of malaria control. Another fish of the same family Poeciliidae, the guppy or *Poecilia* (*Lebistes*) *reticulata* (Peters, 1859), was reported by Sasa *et al.* (1965) in Bangkok as being highly adapted for breeding in polluted waters and an efficient natural enemy of *Culex pipiens fatigans*, the principal vector of the most common type of bancroftian filariasis. Later, a series of extensive investigations were carried out by the author and his colleagues on the use of these and other related species of the fish in the control of mosquitoes and for the treatment of water pollution due to organic matter.

All the poeciliid fishes are indigenous to the Americas, mostly to the tropical and subtropical zones. Being a member of the small fresh water fish of the order Cyprinodontiformes, species of this family differ from others in being ovoviviparous in the mode of reproduction and are apparently adapted for breeding in small pools without vegetation and with little dissolved oxygen content. When introduced

---

* This report was compiled while a Fogarty Scholar-in-Residence, Fogarty International Center, NIH.

into Asian countries, they seem to be capable of breeding in ecological niches where no indigenous Asian fish could survive. The present paper comprises a preliminary report on the use of the poeciliid fishes in Japan and Asia in the basic and applied aspects of environmental sanitation.

THE POECILIID FISHES

The poeciliids are small, fresh or brackish water fish commonly found in tropical and subtropical zones of the Americas. The family Poeciliidae belongs to one of the seven families now recognized in the order Cyprinodontiformes, but differs from the others by being ovoviviparous in the mode of reproduction. The anal fin of the male is usually modified into a sword-like copulating organ called the gonopodium, and the eggs are inseminated and further develop to embryos in the uterus of the females. The mothers give birth to young fish which have reached sizes of over 5 mm in length. Because of this unusual nature, they seem to be capable of breeding in environments such as artificial containers or sewage pools, where no indigenous Asian fish could survive.

An excellent review on morphology, taxonomy and geographic distribution of this fish family was given by Rosen and Bailey (1963) who recognized 3 subfamilies, 21 genera and some 138 species within

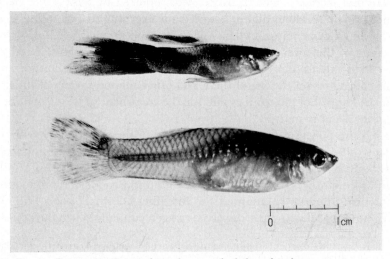

Fig. 1.   Guppy, *Poecilia reticulata:* above: male, below: female.

Poeciliidae. They are all indigenous to the New World, i.e., within the regions from the southern United States, Central America, northern South America, and the West Indies. One of the species commonly called the top minnow, or *Gambusia affinis*, was recognized as an efficient eater of mosquito larvae, and was introduced into other continents from its native land of the southern United States as early as the beginning of this century, mainly for the purpose of malaria control. Several other species of this family, such as the guppy, the moon fish or platy, the sword tail, and the mollies have become popular tropical pet fish and have also been distributed to many countries in the world. Among them, the guppy or *Poecilia reticulata* has been found breeding in wild colonies in some tropical countries in Asia, and was observed by Sasa *et al.* (1965) in Bangkok acting as an excellent natural enemy of *Culex pipiens fatigans*, the principal vector of bancroftian filariasis in the tropical and subtropical countries. Later studies by the same group of workers have demonstrated that this particular fish species is highly adapted for breeding in polluted waters, and might be useful as a biological means of sewage treatment.

Since the fish family Poeciliidae contains a large number of species possibly adapted for breeding in a variety of environments, further studies are needed to explore their use in environmental sanitation. The two species so far extensively investigated by us, the guppy and the top minnow, have been shown to be quite different in certain physiological and ecological aspects, and both have merits and demerits according to the purposes and conditions, as will be discussed later. In Hawaii, for example, the State Health Department uses several species of the poeciliid fish at the same time for the control of mosquito larvae breeding in a variety of environments, and has found that the fish species that breed best differs according to the condition of the water (Nakagawa and Ikeda, 1969). Here, it was also demonstrated that the guppy was best fitted for breeding in the most polluted places, while the distribution of the other fish species according to the reduction of water pollution was the top minnow, the limia and the platy, in that order.

THE TOP MINNOW IN MOSQUITO CONTROL

Among a number of poeciliid fishes, the top minnow or *Gambusia affinis* has been used most extensively for the purpose of mosquito

control. Being a native of the southern United States from Texas to
Florida, it has been introduced and established in most parts of this
country, including California, Michigan and New York. In the
report by Nakagawa and Ikeda (1969), it is stated that a colony of
Gambusia was shipped in 1905 from Texas to Hawaii, where it was
successfully established and distributed to all the principal islands
of Hawaii the next year. Trial introductions of the fish into Europe
mainly for the purpose of malaria control were carried out from the
end of last century, but it is said that these were mostly unsuccessful.
However, the colonies introduced in 1921 into Spain and Italy were
successfully bred, and were further distributed to other European
countries, Africa and southern Asia. A large number of references are
available pertaining to *Gambusia* in relation to the mosquito control,
as reviewed by Gerberich and Laird (1966).

The top minnow is a surface feeder, and is considered to be especially well fitted for feeding on the anopheline larvae which also
stay on the water surface. The fish also eats every small animal in
water that it can swallow, and larvae of culicine mosquitoes are
among its favorite food. However, it is rather doubtful whether the
top minnow has actually contributed to the reduction of malaria in
areas where it was successfully introduced. In our observations, the
top minnow seems to be adapted for breeding in swamps or ditches
containing rather polluted water, but not in natural clean waters
where most malaria vectors breed.

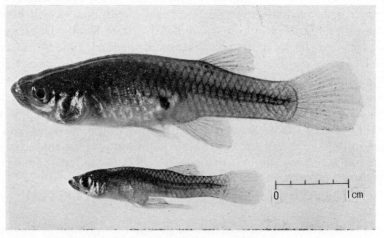

Fig. 2.   Top-Minnow, *Gambusia Affinis;* Above: Female, Below: Male

THE GUPPY AS A NATURAL ENEMY OF FILARIA VECTORS IN SOUTHERN ASIA

The guppy, or *Poecilia* (*Lebistes*) *reticulata* (Peters, 1859), is a popular tropical pet fish, and has been introduced almost all over the world from its native land in areas of tropical South America, including Trinidad and Guiana, especially after World War I. Among guppies, those which were introduced to some South Asian countries have been recognized recently as breeding in wild colonies, mostly in sewage ditches. Such a report was made by Johnson and Soong (1963) from Malaya.

The mosquito *Culex pipiens* s.l. is a common pest as human blood sucker all over the world, and also acts as the principal vector of bancroftian filariasis prevalent in many tropical and subtropical countries. Its larvae breed mainly in sewage pools around houses. The first report on the effectiveness of the guppy as a natural enemy of this particular species of the mosquito was made by Sasa *et al.* (1965), who observed tremendous numbers of the fish breeding in sewage pools in Bangkok. The fish, when introduced into sewage pools where large numbers of the mosquito larvae were found, readily fed on the larvae, and eventually eradicated them within a few months when the fish population reached a certain level. It was also observed that some organophosphorous insecticides, such as fenitrothion, fenthion and ronnel, were effective as larvicides at concentrations of about 0.01 ppm., while their toxicity to the fish was extremely low, being safe to concentrations of about 5 ppm. Therefore, it was suggested that immediately effective and semi-permanent control of the mosquito larvae in such sewage pools could be achieved by simultaneous use of the fish and low-toxicity insecticides.

While visiting Ceylon as WHO consultants to the Anti-Filariasis Campaign, Sasa and Kurihara again discovered a wild colony of the guppy breeding in a sewage ditch in the suburbs of Colombo, and commenced experimental release of the fish into various mosquito breeding habitats. Especially successful was their introduction into abandoned wells and coconut husk pits. Several hundreds of abandoned wells were found in each of the towns in the endemic areas of bancroftian filariasis located along the southwestern coastal belt of this island, which is the most prosperous part of this country. Before the use of the fish, large numbers of laborers were assigned to each town for weekly spraying of malathion in diesel oil, but a single re-

lease of some hundred guppies into each well was usually sufficient
for semi-permanent eradication of the mosquito larvae. The people
were also happy because the well water became clean again, un-
polluted by the diesel oil.

Another successful example was the introduction of the fish into
coconut husk pits. There were many ponds in the endemic areas constructed for the purpose of decaying coconut husks by soaking in
water for several months. From these, the people produced fibers for
mattress and rope. The ponds obviously served as excellent breeding
places for mosquito larvae, but the spraying with diesel oil caused
inhibition of the growth of microorganisms necessary for the fermen-
tation as well as undesired staining of the fiber. The guppies introduced by us into such highly decaying waters largely survived,
reaching enormous population densities in a few months. They not
only eradicated the mosquito breeding, but also helped to produce
good quality fibers as the fish consumed excessively growing microorganisms and stimulated circulation in the water.

The guppy seems to have been established in a number of other
tropical countries, probably all by accidental release by pet breeders.
Kalra et al. (1967) reported on the occurrence of the guppy in sullage
water at Nagpur, India. In a personal communication, Dr. T. Kurihara states that he saw many guppies in sewage ditches around
Djakarta, Indonesia. Dr. J. C. Lien also indicated that he found wild
guppies in a southern district of Taiwan, but the fish could not survive through winter of Taipei. It was introduced recently into
Rangoon, where extensive studies are being carried out by the WHO
assisted Filariasis Control Project (WHO Chronicle, May, 1971).

POECILIIDS ESTABLISHED IN JAPAN

Besides those species which have been imported and are bred in
aquaria as pet fish, at least two poeciliids have been confirmed by us
to be growing in natural habitats of this country, the top minnow and
the guppy. The former was introduced as early as in 1916 for the
purpose of malaria control, while the latter is said to have been imported from about 1930 as a pet fish, but has recently been established
in a number of hot springs.

1. *The top minnow in Japan*
According to the review made by Okada (1957) on the use of fish

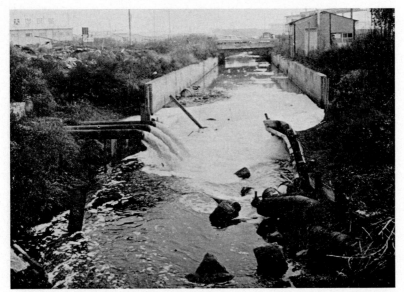

Fig. 3.　A Habitat of the Guppy in Chiba City, Japan; a Stream with Discharging Water at 30°C from a Natural Gas Well.

in malaria control in Japan, the top minnow, *Gambusia affinis* (Baird et Girard, 1853), was shipped by boat from Hawaii to Taiwan in 1911, and was taken further to the mainland of Japan in 1916, first to Koriyama in Nara Prefecture. The colony was successfully bred in one of the goldfish rearing ponds there, and the fish were further transferred to other districts, though no detailed records are available. However, the occurrence of this fish in Japan has been neglected until recently, since the fish was almost absent from the breeding places of *Anopheles sinensis*, the principal vector of malaria in this country. They apparently did not establish in rice paddies and marshes which the malaria vector preferred as breeding sites.

After World War II, the occurrence of the top minnow in areas in and around the world's largest city of Tokyo has begun to attract attention, since large numbers of them were frequently found in highly polluted waters. Surveys have been carried out by members of our department, by Wada, Yamagishi, Shirasaka, and myself since 1964, assisted by sanitary inspectors interested in this field. The fish has been widely found in the Tokyo area, and is obviously the most predominant species even in the suburban zones. There have been a number of sewage pools and abandoned rice paddies untouched in

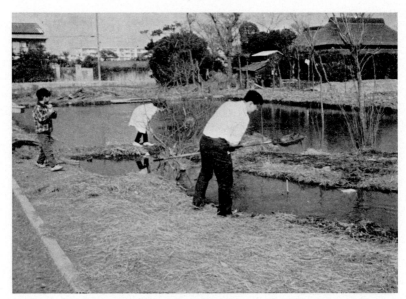

Fig. 4.   A Habitat of the Top-Minnow in Tokyo, a Pond with Sewage Water.

the western and northern out-skirts of this city and there large numbers of *Gamusia* are found breeding. Without them, these pools
would be breeding places of enormous numbers of *Culex pipiens pallens* larvae. They are also found in a number of canals and ditches
connected with the Bay of Tokyo, and even in the bay water near the
piers of the port of Tokyo. The highest sodium chloride concentration
in which the fish have occurred is about 1.5 percent. However, many
of the canals in this city are still free from any fish, as the waters are
too polluted for the survival of even top minnows.

In the summer of 1967, we were informed by the Tokyo International Airport Quarantine Office of the presence of many fish in
ditches of the airport. These were found to be a mixed population of
the top minnow and the indigenous Japanese fish, "Medaka" or
Oryzias latipes. The latter was predominant in the upstream areas of
the ditches between the runways, where the water was rather clean,
while the former was found in pure colonies downstream containing
sewage water from the airport buildings. Their population density
was extremely high, probably because of the absence of any natural
enemies, such as children.

A trial of the use of this fish for a large scale mosquito control
program was carried out by us in the summer of 1968. At that time,

we were requested to assist in organizing a mosquito control project for the city of Tokushima in Shikoku Island by Dr. Okubo and Dr. Sano of the City Health Department, and were considering extensive use of insecticides. A colony of the top minnow collected from the ditch of the Tokyo International Airport was transferred to clean dechlorinated tap water, and as divided into four polyethylene bags, about 100 in each bag, and shipped by air in a cardboard box to Tokushima Airport. They were released into a concrete pond of about 30 m long, 3 m wide and 50 cm in depth, and laboratory animal biscuits were provided every day as their food. The fish started to reproduce immediately thereafter, and the young became mature in about two months. Colonies of the top minnow were further transferred into a number of canals, ditches and swamps of this city from the fall of 1968. The details of this project are being reported by Mr. Sato, who is in charge of the Anti-Mosquito laboratory of Tokushima City. Thus fish newly introduced into this area have already established large colonies in almost every water where they can breed, and have contributed a great deal to reducing the pest mosquitoes, including *Culex pipiens pallens*, that carry filariasis. The city of Tokushima is built on a low delta of a big river, as is Bangkok, and thus is surrounded by swamps, canals and ditches difficult to drain. The top minnow was again shown here to be very useful under such environmental conditions. There are acres of swamps in the suburbs of this city that used to be breeding places of a variety of mosquito species (*Culex pipiens pallens, C. tritaeniorhynchus, Aedes dorsalis, Anopheles sinensis*, etc.), but these have been mostly replaced by large numbers of the predatory fish, *Gambusia*.

2. *The guppy in Japan*

The history of introduction of the guppy into Japan is quite different from that of the top minnow. It is said that these fish were first imported into this country in about 1930, and became popular after the World War II as a tropical pet fish. Even now, large numbers of them are imported every year from Singapore and Hongkong by commercial dealers. It is said that it is much cheaper to import them from tropical countries than to try mass breeding under artificial heat through the winter of Japan. All the guppies now available in Japan are more or less artificially selected "fancy" strains, and the males are colorful and long-tailed, even those found as wild colonies in hot spring areas.

According to our previous experience, all the guppies so far tested by us have been incapable of surviving through the winter in the temperate zone, although trials are in progress for selecting cold-resistant strains. The known northern limit in Asia at which the fish can survive through winter under natural conditions is Hongkong and southern Taiwan. All the guppy colonies we sent from Tokyo to our branch laboratory in southern Amami Island near Okinawa have so far failed to survive through the winter season, where the average temperature in February is about 10°C.

It was therefore a surprise to us when we were informed in 1964 that the guppies occurred as wild populations in some rural districts near Tokyo. It eventually became clear that all the habitats of the wild guppies so far known are in the hot spring areas, and they survive through the winter downstream from the hotsprings where the water temperature is kept above 20°C all through the year. In a monthly survey carried out by Yamagishi et al. (1966) in Tokura Spa and in another monthly survey carried out by us in Rendaiji Spa, the guppies were found to be breeding almost everywhere during the summer season, including the hot spring ditches, streams, rice paddies and swamps, but were seen hibernating only in the warm waters during the season from December to April. Such hot spring ditches take overflow waters from bath tubs of hotels and also highly polluted sewage waters, and the dissolved oxygen contents are usually very low, sometimes below 2 ppm. The fish seem to be protected from attack of indigenous carnivorous fishes by taking shelter in such warm and polluted waters.

The guppies have so far been found in Tokura-Kamiyamada Spa, Asama Spa and Kamisuwa Spa of Nagano Prefecture, Uchigo Spa of Fukushima Prefecture, Rendaiji Spa of Shizuoka Prefecture, and Beppu Spa of Oita Prefecture. In our survey carried out in April 1971 in the Uchigo area, it was confirmed that both the guppy and the top minnow were breeding in a river of about 70 m in width. Hot water pumped up from nearby coal mines was continuously discharged into this river at a rate of 100 tons per min, and the water temperature of the river near the discharging site was as high as 41°C. Both guppies and top minnows were found actively swimming in such a hot environment. The two species in the same river were, however, found to be more or less separated as populations; the colonies of the guppy were seen mostly in shallow and polluted places with shelters, such as spots where garbage collects, while the top minnows were seen swimming rather freely in the streams. In this town, there were also a number of highly polluted sewage pools containing hot spring water, but these were inhabited only by guppies. We were told from the manager of a hotel that the guppies had become established from a colony bred in a pond from about 1966, when the town was flooded by a typhoon. However, no explanation could be given as to why the top minnow had reached this town, located about 400 km north of Tokyo.

Trials to release the guppy into other hot spring areas have been carried out occasionally by members of our laboratory. In March 1968, for example, a team composed of myself, Shirasaka and Wada drove a car loaded with guppies bred in our laboratory to the Izu Peninsula, inspected about 20 hot spring towns, and released guppies in adequate sites. Many of the hot springs were located on steep slopes, and there were no possible breeding places for them. Promising sites were found in Shirata Spa, Mine Spa, Shimokamo Spa, Shuzenji Spa, Nagaoka Spa and Hatage Spa, and several colonies composed of about 50 fishes each were released. In subsequent surveys carried out in the same areas, successful establishment as wild colonies was seen in only two instances, at Shimokamo and Hatage. In the former, the fish released by us became a large colony in one of the streams, but died out the same winter when the water temperature rose as high as 60°C. In Hatage, the guppies were released into a swamp where large numbers of indigenous Japanese fish were already seen breeding together with natural enemies such as crayfish and bullfrogs, but the guppies have become visible in enormous numbers since May 1970.

Trials for mass-breeding of the guppy utilizing hot springs have also been carried out, one of the most successful of which is a project sponsored by the Kagoshima Prefecture Health Department and supervised by Mr. Kawagoe of Ibusuki Health Center. Six large concrete pools originally constructed for the breeding of "Suppon" (snapping turtle) but abandoned later were utilized, and fancy strains of the guppies released in 1968 were bred in millions the next year by providing about one kg of a standard fish food (for rearing carp) every day. Hot spring water was introduced into the ponds during the winter time to keep the temperature above 25°C, and the guppies thus bred to enormous numbers and were supplied to municipalities the next spring where they were released in adequate numbers into various mosquito breeding places.

Another interesting habitat for the guppy where it can survive throughout the year is the sewage pools under big buildings and subways in large cities, where the water temperature is kept warm through the winter by artificial heating. A mosquito called *Culex pipiens molestus* has been recognized to be breeding in enormous numbers in these dark pools, and has become a nuisance to the city people, even during the winter season. In our experience, guppies released into these basement sewage pools have been mostly found breeding in successive generations, and are effective as a predator of the mosquito larvae. A colony released in a newly constructed building in Kofu City in 1968 were confirmed to have survived through two winters in the basement, and the building became free of the mosquito larvae.

An unusual habitat of the guppy associated with modern industrialization and urbanization was found in a satellite city of Tokyo. There is a deep well constructed for digging underground natural gas near Chiba City, and about 20 ton per min of underground water with a temperature of about 30°C is continuously discharged into a stream called the Yoshikawa River. The stream runs through the busiest part of the city for about 6 km as a canal, until it combines with a larger river. The guppies were found to be breeding in large numbers all through this stream which becomes highly polluted as it passes through the city. A monthly survey has been commenced since this was discovered in November 1970 by members of our department and the Chiba Prefecture Health Laboratories. The water temperature of the canal was kept at 25°C or higher during the winter season through the downstream area from the site of intake of the well water, and tremendous numbers of the guppies were found in this range of several km. From June, when the water temperature of the natural surface waters rises above 25°C, the guppies were seen spreading upstream and into the connecting ditches or rice paddies for a range of over 5 km.

Such a finding suggests the possibility of mass breeding of the guppies by utilizing excess heat produced by various industries, such as the electric power plants, chemical or pharmaceutical plants, and so forth. As long as such excess heat is available, the guppies may be useful as a part of the sewage disposal system for the removal of organic contaminants.

LABORATORY OBSERVATIONS

Laboratory studies have been carried out and some are in progress on comparative physiology, reproduction, larvivorous activity, and relation to water pollution of the poeciliid fishes. A part of the results of our experiments were reported by Sasa *et al.* (1965), Yamagishi *et al.* (1966, 1967) and Sasa (1970), and are in preparation. The following is a summary of our observations, including some unpublished data.

Predation on mosquito larvae

Both the guppy and the top minnow are efficient feeders on mosquito larvae. Even the newborn young can feed on first and second stage larvae. The amount of larvae consumed by the fish differs according to size and sex, temperature of water and presence of other food. In the observations made by Sasa *et al.* (1965) in Bangkok, the numbers of fourth instar larvae of *Culex pipiens fatigans* eaten per day per fish was 31.6 for female guppies and 19.2 for males (average of 10 fishes each, for one week). In the experiments carried out by Yamagishi (1966) with guppies collected at a hot spring, the females (70–581 mg in body weight) consumed 21–91 mg or 10–36 fourth instar larvae of *Culex pipiens pallens* per day on the average, at 25°C, while the amount of consumption decreased with temperature decreases to 30°C, 20°C, and 15°C. In another observation carried out by Sato *et al.* (1970) at a water temperature of 27°C, the numbers of fourth instar larvae consumed each by 15 adults of the guppy and the top minnow per week were 207.9 (340-155) and 228.0 (112-414), respectively, or the daily averages of 29.7 and 32.6.

It should be also noted here that more effective control of mosquito larvae may be achieved by simultaneous use of biological and chemical measures than their individual applications. Sasa *et al.* (1965) have shown that some organophosphorous insecticides available to us, such as fenitrothion, fenthion and ronnel, kill the mosquito larvae at a level lower than 0.01 ppm, but are toxic to the fish only the level reaches about 5 ppm (Table 1). The insecticides sprayed into a mosquito breeding place may be effective to kill all the larvae but the effects are always transient and the operation must be repeated at certain intervals. On the other hand, relatively small numbers of guppies released into breeding places are usually not sufficient to clean up the larvae, and it usually requires two or more months until

Table 1. Relative Toxicity of Insecticides to Larvae of *Culex pipiens*
fatigans, *Aedes aegypti* and to a Mosquito Eating Fish Guppy, *Lebistes*
reticulatus
(Provisional estimates of lethal concentrations in ppm with the respective percent-mortality, based on laboratory experiments at
28–30°C in 24 hours exposure, for wild colonies collected at Din
Dang, southeast Bangkok).

Insecticides	*fatigans*		*aegypti*	*Lebistes*		Safety index
	LC 95	LC 50	LC 50	LC 50	LC 05	
1. p-p' DDT	1.5	0.3	0.2	0.05	0.01	0.007
2. tech. DDT	1.0	0.2	0.2	0.06	0.01	0.01
3. Lindane	0.6	0.1	0.05	0.5	0.3	0.5
4. Chlordane	1.6	0.3	0.2	0.3	0.1	0.06
5. Dieldrin	0.16	0.04	0.03	0.02	0.005	0.03
6. Diazinon	0.05	0.03	0.07	0.3	0.2	4.0
7. Malathion	0.08	0.03	0.05	1.0	0.3	4.0
8. Sumithion	0.006	0.003	0.004	5.5	4.5	750.
9. Fenthion	0.006	0.003	0.004	5.0	4.0	670.
10. Ronnel	0.008	0.005	0.04	2.5	1.5	200.
11. Dichlorvos	0.05	0.025	0.03	7.0	3.0	60.
12. Trichlorfon	0.06	0.03	0.07	10.0	4.0	67.

Safety index: LC-05 (or maximum safety concentration) against *Lebistes* divided
by LC-95 (or minimum effective concentration) against *fatigans*.
After Sara, *et al.* (1965)

population density of the fish reaches an effective level. In our semi-
natural experiments carried out outdoors in Tokyo, it was shown that
immediate and permanent eradication of mosquito breeding could
be achieved for tanks containing 150 liter of septic water by adding
10 couples of guppies and 1.5 ml of 10% emulsion of fenitrothion at
the same time. The insecticide killed all the mosquito larvae which
were already present, and the fish consumed all mosquito egg rafts or
first stage larvae subsequently deposited in the tanks. As stated
above, the average number of fourth stage larvae eaten by one fish
per day is about 30, but the same fish consumes about 1,000 eggs or
first stage larvae. Therefore, efficiency in control of mosquito breeding can be greatly enhanced by the integrated method.

Reproduction and laboratory breeding
Guppies are easily bred in small aquaria, as every pet breeder

knows. In the observations by Yamagishi *et al.* (1967) with the colony breeding in Tokura Spa, the numbers of offspring produced by a female at one birth varied from 8 to 52, the number being closely related to the body length of the mother. The growth of the young under adequate conditions is very fast, and they reach over 20 mm at 25°C in two months, giving birth to the next generation from about the 60th day. The first batch of young produced by the female is usually small in number, about 10 on the average, but they gradually increase as the mother becomes larger. The interval between births is from 30 to 41 days. The parents usually do not eat the young when kept in a container by themselves, but predation on the young by adult fish occurs when the population density of an aquarium becomes very high.

The top minnows, on the other hand, have been found to be extremely difficult to breed in aquaria. When a colony collected in the field is kept in a container of 20 liter or larger, the population never increases as in the case of guppies, but gradually decreases until a big female is left alone. If a pregnant female is kept singly in a container, she may produce young, but subsequent births are rare even when a male is added. This species of fish seems to require a certain space in the environment for reproduction. Successful breeding of top minnows could be achieved in our laboratory only when they were released into pools with a minimum size of 130 cm length, 70 cm width and 35 cm depth. In one of our observations, 5 couples each of the top minnow and the guppy were released into four such pools, two pools for each species, at the end of April, 1967. The pools were harvested in November of the same year. The numbers of the top minnow collected were 157 and 126 respectively, while 3,742 and 3,363 guppies were found in pools of the same size.

Resistance to temperature

Under laboratory conditions, both the guppies and the top minnows could not survive at water temperatures above 36°C, though in nature we have seen especially acclimatized populations living in water of 41°C at Uchigo. The resistance to low temperature differs greatly between the two species; the lowest temperature at which the guppies could survive was roughly 13°C in our observations with various strains, while the top minnows could stand temperatures as low as 4°C in the laboratory, and all the outdoor colonies kept in pools 1.3 m long, 0.7 m wide and 0.35 m deep have survived through freezing temperatures for four winters in Tokyo. All the guppy colonies kept outdoors or in a room without heating died during December when the temperature dropped to near 10°C. When the colonies kept at 20°C are exposed to a gradual drop of temperature at a speed of −1°C per min., the guppies start to die from about 15°C, and all follow suit at 10°C. Therefore, mixed colonies of the two species such as that collected at Uchigo could be clearly distinguished by exposing them to 10°C; at that temperature those still surviving were all top minnows.

Relation to organic pollution

In our field observations, both the guppies and top minnows in Japan and South Asia have been seen breeding mostly in polluted waters with relatively high BOD (Biological Oxygen Demand) and low DO (Dissolved Oxygen content). They seem to be more adapted or tolerant to pollution from organic matter than most indigenous fish, and to prefer to stay in such an environment. However, it is not easy to find out what factors are essentially involved in their tolerance and preference. A series of investigations are in progress, mainly by Dr. T. Kurihara, for elucidation of such a relationship. The following is a summary of our preliminary studies.

In general, these poeciliid fishes are tolerant to pollution from nutrient substances (especially protein and carbohydrates), but not necessarily to chemical pollution (free chlorine, heavy metal, cyanide compounds, etc). For example, both guppies and top minnows were all killed within four hours when released into tap water containing 0.5 ppm of free chlorine, and did not survive longer than two hours at 0.6 ppm, though both tolerated concentrations of 0.3 ppm or lower.

In most of our experiments, standard septic water was prepared by adding a certain amount of dry powdered laboratory animal food to tap water in a room regulated at 25°C. When 10 g of the food is added to 10 liter of water in a glass container, the dissolved oxygen value (DO) drops gradually and becomes almost zero ppm (i.e. not detectable by usual chemical or electric measures) within 6 hours, and remains so for more than a week. However, the guppies released in such septic water usually survive very well as long as the water surface is exposed to the air. Under such conditions, all the guppies come up to the water surface for breathing, and occasionally dive into the bottom for a few seconds or longer to take food (the decaying matter and microorganisms in the sediment). When certain numbers of the guppies are released into such septic waters, such as 20 to 50 adults per 10 liter of water, the fish eventually clean up the decaying matter and the DO value of the water rises to certain level within a few days. It would otherwise remain undetectable for several weeks. The guppies in a natural environment are also considered to be the sweeper or cleaner of sewage waters.

However, there is a limit to the pollution the guppies can tolerate, though this may be much higher than for other fish. For example, septic water produced by adding 10 g of animal food powder per 10 liter is usually well tolerated, but dosages of 20 g or higher cause lethal effects on the guppies, usually after 3 or 4 days, when the water becomes highly septic and causes a strong smell. Since the DO value becomes undetectable as early as within 24 hours, the lack of oxygen in the water is presumed not to be the cause of their death. In Dr. Kurihara's preliminary investigations, the toxicity of such septic waters against the guppies is closely related to the concentration of free H_2S which becomes maximum at the stage when its concentration is the highest. The increase in free ammonia takes place somewhat later. In his observation, lethal concentrations of free H_2S and NH_3 are 2 ppm and 18 ppm respectively, and thus he suspects that the former could be the principal factor that kills the guppies under these conditions. Top minnows exposed to similar conditions are usually less tolerant to pollution.

SUMMARY

A review was made of our field and laboratory investigations on the biology of two poeciliid fish imported to and established in Asia, with emphasis on their significance as natural enemies of mosquitoes and with relation to water pollution.

The guppy, *Poecilia reticulata*, is a native of tropical South America but was found in 1954 in Bangkok acting as an effective natural enemy of mosquito larvae, especially *Culex pipiens fatigans*. It has subsequently been utilized in effective measures in the control of filariasis in Ceylon and elsewhere. This fish was found also to be adapted for breeding in highly polluted waters, and is effective in removing decaying matter when it reaches a certain population density. It is, however, incapable of surviving the low temperatures of the winter in temperate zones. In Japan, it has been found breeding in wild colonies in several hot spring areas, and successful mass breeding could be achieved by utilizing natural hot springs. The fish was also effective in the control of *Culex pipiens molestus* in the basements of buildings and subways, where the sewage water is kept warm throughout the year.

The top minnow, *Gambusia affinis*, was imported in 1916 for the purpose of malaria control, and has been found established in large numbers in canals and bay waters in and around Tokyo. It also breeds mainly in polluted waters and acts as an excellent mosquito-eater but is less tolerant of pollution than the guppy. A colony was introduced into Tokushima city of Shikoku Island in 1968 for the purpose of mosquito control and has been successfully established in many sewage ditches and swamps. The top minnow can survive through the freezing temperature of winter in Japan, but has difficulty breeding in small artificial containers.

REFERENCES

Burton, G. J. (1960). Studies on the bionomics of vectors which transmit filariasis in India. IV. Observations on larvivorous activities of various fishes in filarial areas of Kerala State, South India. *Ind. J. Malariol.*, **14**, 131.

Gordon, M. (1960). Guppies. A guide to the selection, care and breeding of the guppies. Jersey City, N.J.

Johnson, D. S. and Soong, M. H. H. (1963). The fate of introduced freshwater fish in Malaya. Proc. XVI Intern. Congr. Zool. **1**, 246, Washington, D.C.

Kalra, N. L., Watal, B. L. and Raghavan, N. G. S. (1967). Occurrence of larvivorous fish *Lebistes reticulatus* (Peters) breeding in sullage water at Nagpur-India. *Bull. Indian Soc. Mal. Com. Dis.*, **4**(3), 253.

Makino, S. (1963). Tropical Fishes (in Japanese), 127 pp., Hoikusha, Tokyo.

Gerberich, J. B. and Laird, M. (1966). Annoted bibliography of papers relating to control of mosquitos by the use of fish. (Revised and enlarged to 1965). WHO/EBL/66.71 (mimeographed, 107 pp.); (1968) Bibliography of papers relating to the control of mosquitos by the use of fish, FAO Fisheries Tech. Paper, No. 75.

Nakagawa, P. Y. and Ikeda, R. M. (1969). Biological control of mosquitoes with larvivorous fish in Hawaii. WHO/VBC/69.173 (mimeographed, 25 pp.)

Okada, Y. (1957). "Fishes as natural enemies of malaria mosquitoes, with special reference to the top minnow." (in Japanese) Kankyo Eisei, No. **10**, 6–13.

Rosen, D. E. and Bailey, R. M. (1963). The poeciliid fishes (Cyprinodontiformes), their structure, zoogeography, and systematics. *Bull. Amer. museum Nat. Sci. Hist.*, 126 Art. 1.

Sasa, M. *et al.* (1965). Studies on mosquitoes and their natural enemies in Bangkok, Pt. 2. Insecticide suceptibility of the larvae of *Culex pipiens igans, Aedes aegypti* and the mosquito eating fish *Lebistes reticulatus*. Pt. 3. Observations on a mosquito eating fish "guppy" or *Lebistes reticulatus* breeding in polluted waters. *Japan. J. Exp. Med.*,

35, (1), 51.

Sasa, M. (1970). "Biological measures in environmental sanitation, with special reference to the use of poeciliid fishes." (in Japanese) Gakujutsu Geppo **23** (10), 601.

Sasa, M. (1971). "The use of poeciliid fishes in environmental sanitation." (in Japanese) Baioteku, Kodansha, **2** (8), 627–632.

Sato, H. *et al.* (1970). "Comparative studies on the two poeciliid fishes, *Lebistes reticulatus* and *Gambusia affinis*, as natural enemies of mosquito larvae." (in Japanese) Eisei Dobutsu (*Japan. J. Sanitary Zool.*,) **21** (2), 25 (abstract).

World Health Organization (1971). Vector Control. *WHO Chronicle*, **25**(5), 199.

Yamagishi, H. *et al.* (1966). Ecological studies on guppy, *Lebistes reticulatus* Peters. 1. Acclimatized guppy in the waters of hot spring in Japan (in Japanese).

Eisei Dobutsu (*Japan. J. Sanitary Zool.*), **17**(1), 48; II. Experiments on predation of mosquito larvae by guppies (in Japanese). *J. Fac. Sci. Shinshu Univ.*, **1**(2), 79; (1967). III. On the guppy population acclimatized in a water of Tokura-Kamiyamada Spa. *Japan. J. Ecology*, **17**(5), 206.

Schistosoma Infection among Dairy Cows in the Tone River Basin in Chiba Prefecture

M. Yokogawa,* M. Sano,* S. Kojima,* K. Araki,*
K. Ogawa,* T. Yamada,** A. Shimotokube,** T. Iijima,**
K. Higuchi** and S. Hayasaka**

*Department of Parasitology, School of Medicine,
Chiba University, Chiba, Japan
**Chiba Prefectural Institute of Animal Health,
Narita, Chiba, Japan

INTRODUCTION

Very recently, Nakano (1970) reported that an endemic disease with manifestations similar to those of schistosomiasis japonica was present among dairy cows pastured on the dry bed of the Tone River in Chiba Prefecture. He assumed that these cows must have been infected while grazing on the river bed. According to him, the main sysmptoms of the disease were dysentery, anorexia, weight loss and hypertrophy of the rectal wall. He also reported that he found the characteristic eggs of *Schistosoma japonicum* in bloody mucus in the stool. However, he failed to find the snail intermediate host of *Schistosoma japonicum* in the grazing areas.

Upon reviewing the report of Nakano, the authors agreed that a great danger to the inhabitants of the neighborhood would exist if the disease found among the dairy cows was actually a result of infection with *Schistosoma japonicum*. Thus, they initiated an intensive survey for schistosomiasis, the results of which are reported here. In Narita city and Shimofusa Town, assumed to be areas where the disease was endemic, blood was collected from dairy cows for serological screening tests with complement fixation (CF) and circum oval precipitin (COP) tests, and a search was made for *Oncomelania nosophora*, the intermediate host of *Schistosoma japonicum*, on the bed of the Tone River.

MATERIALS AND METHODS

A total of 296 dairy cows from the suspected areas were surveyed; 181 at Tatsudai (I) in Narita City and 115 at Kobuke, Takaoka, Namegawa and Shinkawa (II) in Shimofusa Town. A group of 81 dairy cows which had never been pastured in a river bed, from Nagoya (III) in Shimofusa Town several kilometers away from the river, served as controls (Fig. 1).

The CF test employed was the same as that developed by Yokogawa and Awano (1956) for human serum for paragonimiasis. The antigen was a 1:4000 dilution of a Veronal buffered saline extract of adult worms of *S. japonicum* (VBS antigen). A reaction of 1:10 or greater in a 50% hemolysis end point titration was considered as positive.

The COP test of Oliver-Gonzalez (1954) was used, and the eggs of *S. japonicum* were collected by the digestion technique following the modified technique of Yokogawa and Sano (1966).

Stools were collected for 5 consecutive days from cows which exhibited positive reactions in either serologic test, and examined for

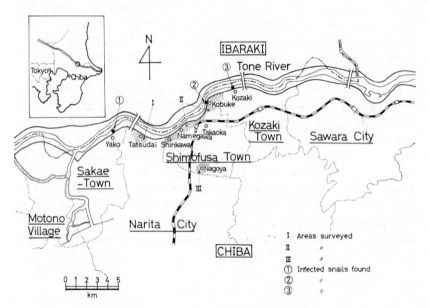

Fig. 1.   Detailed Map of Tone River Area in Chiba Prefecture.

Schistosoma eggs with the AMS-III centrifugation technique and by the miracidium hatching test.

An intensive search was conducted for the snail host in all suitable habitat areas along the Tone River bed from the area of Yako on the western side to Kozaki on the eastern side (Fig. 1).

RESULTS

The results of the CF and COP screening tests are summarized in Table 1. In the Tatsudai area (I), of 181 cows 3 (1.7%) showed positive CF reactions, and 8 (4.4%) positive COP reactions. Two of the CF positive cows also had a positive reaction in the COP test, but one had a positive reaction in this test only, so there was a total of 9 cows (5.0%) with a positive reaction in either test. In the Kobuke and other areas (II), 30 out of 115 cows (26.1%) had a positive COP reaction, and 8 of these also had a positive CF reaction. Among the 81 cows of the control group from the Nagoya area (III), no positive serological test results were seen.

The results of stool examinations on the serologically positive cows are presented in Table 2. Five of 9 (55.6%) cows examined from Tatsudai (I) were demonstrated to be positive either for *Schistosoma*

Table 1. Results of Screening Test for *Schistosoma* Infections in Dairy-cows with COP-and CF-Tests

Areas		No. exam.	No. (%) positive		
			CF-Test	COP-Test	Total
I	Tatsudai	181	3(1.7%)	8(4.4%)	9**(5.0%)
II	Kobuke & others	115	8(7.0%)	30(26.1%)	30**(26.1%)
III	Nagoya*	81	0	0	0

  * Cows have never been pastured in river bed.
 ** Total no. of cows positive by either CF or COP.

Table 2. Results of Stool Examination for *Schistosoma* Eggs or Miracidium in Dairy cows with Positive CF-or COP-Tests

Areas	No. exam.	No. (%) positive for eggs or miracidium
I. Tatsudai	9	5 (55.6%)
II. Kobuke & others	30	15 (50.0%)
Total	39	20 (51.3%)

M. YOKOGAWA ET AL.

eggs or hatched miracidia. Similarly, 15 of 30 (50.0%) cows from Kobuke and others (II) were positive; thus, 20 of 39 cows from the suspected area were confirmed to be infected with *S. japonicum*. With the AMS-III centrifugation method, eggs were found in 15 of the 20 proved cases, while in 18 of the 20 proved cases miracidia were hatched.

The correlation between the serologic tests and stool examinations is shown in Table 3. Of 10 cows with positive reactions in both tests, 10 (100%) were infected as confirmed by stool examination, while 35.7% of those positive by the COP alone had positive stool examinations. The one cow positive by CF only also had negative stool results.

The snail intermediate host (*Oncomelania nosophora*) of *Schistosoma japonicum* was encountered in considerable numbers in the Tone river bed in the areas where the infected dairy cows were pastured. These areas were damp, with small pools scattered over the low areas and they appeared to be ideal habitats for this snail. As indicated in Table 4, a total of 273 snails were examined for cercariae of *S. japonicum*. High infection rates were seen in snails from Yako (27.5%), Kobuke (52.3%) and Kozaki (14.0%), with an overall average of 37.0% infected.

Table 3.   Correlation between Immuno-Serological Tests and
Stool Examinations

Immuno. Tests	No. exam.	No. (%) positive for eggs or miracidium
CF-T + COP-T +	10	10 (100%)
CF-T + COP-T −	1	0
CF-T − COP-T +	28	10 (35.7%)

Table 4.   The Incidence of *S. japonicum* Infection in *Oncomelania nosophora* Collected from the bed of Tone River

Areas	No. exam.	No. (%) infected
1—Yako	91	25 (27.5%)
2—Kobuke	132	69 (52.3%)
3—Kozaki	50	7 (14.0%)
Total	273	101 (37.0%)

DISCUSSION

According to Nakano (1970), dairy cows were first introduced into this area of Chiba Prefecture from Hokkaido in 1955 and the number increased rapidly sometime around 1962. All the cows pastured on the dry bed of the Tone River were dairy cows and none were draft animals.

It was in 1914 that *O. nosophora* was first found on the Tone river bed (Takagi, 1914; Miyagawa and Mizobuchi, 1916). In 1947, Wright *et al.* (1947) carried out a field survey for schistosomiasis in the Tone river basin where schistosomiasis japonica was prevalent. They reported that, although few persons infected with schistosomiasis japonica were found in Sakura and Sawara areas along the Tone River in Chiba Prefecture, that they failed to find *Oncomelania* snails in the dry bed of the Tone.

Olivier (1948) reported that he found *O. nosophora* several miles above Toride, Ibaragi Prefecture, on the Tone River north of Chiba Prefecture. Ritchie *et al.* (1953) reported that they collected *O. nosophora* in 13 of 27 areas where they searched for snails on the dry river bed on the Chiba Prefecture side, but that only 2 out of 15 *O. nosophora* found in Kobuke were infected with the cercariae of *S. japonicum*.

In more recent years, only Komiya (1955) has reported *O. nosophora* snails found on the left bank of the Naka River, a tributary of the Tone, in Saitama Prefecture. No *O. nosophora* found in the Tone River basin has been reported for the past 18 years. The Kobuke area (Shimofusa Town) where the authors found *Oncomelania* snails in the present study is the locality where Ritchie *et al.* (1953) made their extensive survey. As mentioned above, only 15 *Oncomelania* snails were found during the survey of Ritchie, *et al.*, whereas innumerable *O. nosophora* were found in the present study. The very high percentage infected with *S. japonicum* is most remarkable. The definitive hosts of *S. japonicum* in nature, other than humans, can be cows, horses, dogs, cats, rats, and several other mammals; but in Japan, cows used as draft animals in agriculture were hitherto the most important reservoir host. It is a notable new development revealed by the present study that imported dairy cows, and not native cows, used as work animals in agriculture were an important source of *Schistosoma* infection.

The screening methods used to detect *Schistosoma* infections in cows yielded results which correspond closely to those obtained with mass surveys for human schistosomiasis by the authors (1970). This indicates that the methods employed for the present study are also applicable and effective for mass surveys on cows.

It is apparent that the COP test is much more sensitive and effective than the CF-test as a screening method for *Schistosoma* infection in cows. It can also safely be said that the CF-test may show false negative reactions, although a positive CF-test reaction may strongly suggest present infection.

The inhabitants of the areas have not yet been clinically evaluated for schistosomiasis japonica. However, those who have frequented the river bed have naturally been exposed to the danger of being infected, and surveys for schistosomiasis among the inhabitants of the areas are now in progress.

SUMMARY

Recently Nakano (1970) reported that a peculiar disease resembling schistosomiasis was prevalent among dairy cows pastured on the bed of the Tone River in Chiba Prefecture. He described the main features of the disease as bloody, mucous diaorrhea, hypertrophy of the rectal wall, and eggs resembling *S. japonicum* in the feces.

Because of the obvious hazard to humans in the area, the present survey was conducted to determine the extent and severity of the focus. A total of 296 dairy cows were screened serologically using complement fixation and circum-oval precipitin tests. Cows from an area several kilometers from the river served as a control group. Feces from serologically positive cows were examined for *Schistosoma* eggs by AMS-III centrifugation and miracidia hatching techniques.

Among cows pastured on the river bed, 9 of 181 (5.0%) in one locality, and 30 of 115 (26.1%) in another showed positive reactions in either of the two tests. Fecal examinations of the 39 serologically positive cows showed eggs or miracidia of *S. japonicum* in 20 (51.3%). No cows showing positive reaction in serological tests were found in the control group. An intensive search for the snail intermediate host revealed large populations of *Oncomelania nosphora* in river bed areas used to pasture the infected cows. Extremely high infection rates were found, cercariae being demonstrated in 37% of 273 snails examined, with infection rates over 50% in some areas.

REFERENCES

Kashiwado, T., Nakamura, T., Akiyama, T., Shikata, I., Fuse, Y., Hirokawa, S., Ishijima, F., Beniya, S., Takagi, T., Mihashi, S. and Enokizawa, M. (1927). Outline of clinical studies on schistosomiasis japonica occurring in Sakura area, Chiba Prefecture. *Jour. Chiba Med. Soc.*, **5**, 1473. (in Japanese)

Komiya, Y. (1955). On schistosomiasis japonica in Saitama Prefecture. *Chiryo Yakuho*, **553**, 18. (in Japanese)

Miyagawa, M. and Mizobuchi, T. (1914). On the distribution of schistosomiasis japonica in Ibaragi Prefecture. *Iji Shinbun*, **893**, 1. (in Japanese)

Nakano, M. (1970). An occurrence of schistosomiasis-like disease in cows. A peculiar disease of the rectal wall of cows pastured in a river bed. *Kachiku Shinryo*, **86**, 23. (in Japanese)

Olivier, L. (1948). A note on schistosomiasis in eastern Japan. *Amer. J. Trop. Med.*, **28**, 867.

Oliver-Gonzalez, J. (1954). Anti-egg precipitin in the serum of human infected with *Schistosoma mansoni*. *J. Inf. Dis.*, **96**, 86.

Ritchie, L. S., Hunter, G. W. III, Kaufman, E. H., Pan, C., Yokogawa, M., Nagano, K. and Szewczack, J. T. (1953). Parasitological studies in the far east. VIII. An epidemiologic study on the Tone river area, Japan. *Jap. J. Med. Sci. & Biol.*, **6**, 33.

Takagi, O. (1914). On schistosomiasis japonica in Takano-mura, Kita-Soma-gun, Ibaragi Prefecture. *Jap. J. Bacteriol.*, **228**, 30. (in Japanese)

Wright, W. H., McMullen, D. B., Bennett, H. J., Bauman, P. M. and Iugalls, J. W. (1947). The epidemiology of schistosomiasis japonica in the Philippines and Japan. III. Surveys of endemic areas of schistosomiasis japonica in Japan. *Amer. J. Trop. Med.*, **27**, 417.

Yokogawa, M. (1970). Schistosomiasis in Japan. Recent Advances in Researches and Schistosomiasis in Japan. University of Tokyo Press, 231–255.

Yokogawa, M. and Awano, R. (1956). On the complement-fixation test for paragonimiasis. Relation between the intradermal test and the complement-fixation test. *Nihon Iji Shimpo*, **1703**, 27. (in Japanese)

Yokogawa, M. and Sano, M. (1966). Immunosero-diagnosis of schistosomiasis japonica. II. Isolation technique of the *Schistosoma* eggs from tissue for circumoval precipitation test. *Jap. J. Parasit.*, **15**, 394. (in Japanese)

Epidemiological Study of Schistosomiasis Japonica with Special Reference to Distribution of Intermediate Host Snails in an Endemic Area

T. Ishizaki,* Y. Ito,* Y. Hosaka* and H. Kutsumi**

* Department of Parasitology, National Institute of Health, Tokyo, Japan
** Department of Endemic Diseases, Yamanashi Prefectural Hygiene Laboratory, Kofu, Japan

INTRODUCTION

The occurrence of a snail-transmitted parasitic disease is usually limited to an area in which the intermediate host snail can live. Schistosomiasis japonica is still found in Japan and its infection rate among the inhabitants varies with the village in endemic areas (Okabe, 1938a, b; 1939). When a family in an endemic area is examined as a unit in an epidemiological investigation of the disease, there is a tendency of frequent occurrence of the disease among the members of one family. This fact may serve as a clue to where the actual infection occurs.

The present study was intended to determine the actual correlation between the occurrence of the disease in a patient and distribution of the intermediate host snail, *Oncomelania nosophora*, in an endemic area. Data obtained from family histories were also utilized in the study.

MATERIALS AND METHODS

1. *Subjects*

Seventeen families were selected on the basis of clinical examinations which were carried out in an endemic area of schistosomiasis, Ryuo Town in Yamanashi Prefecture, Japan. These families were engaged in farming and their ricefields were located in the endemic area.

The families were divided into three groups according to the number of cases in a family: 1) highly infected families in which there are 2 or more (egg-positive) cases, 2) moderately infected families in

[95]

which there is one egg-positive case, and 3) uninfected families. In the first group were 31 persons from 7 highly infected families; in the second, 18 persons from 4 moderately infected families, and in the third, 20 from 6 uninfected families.

2. *Family history*

As the symptoms of *S. japonicum* infection were common in this area, family histories including those of the parents of the house holder were examined for cirrhosis with ascites. Survey participants were questioned on chronic disorders especially on schistosomiasis and results of previous fecal examinations and skin tests for schistosome infection. Inquiry was also made about their farming habit of going barefoot, the use of nightsoil in their rice fields, and the rearing of cattle or other domestic animals.

3. *Fecal examination*

A fecal examination was carried out in each of 1 g of fecal specimen by means of the modified MIFC method (Ota and Sato, 1957). This examination was performed 3 times on a person at 7-day intervals.

4. *Skin test*

The antigen used in the test is an acid-soluble protein fraction prepared from adult *S. japonicum* by Melcher's method (1943). The standard antigen contains 30 μg of protein nitrogen per ml. Two-hundredths ml of the standard antigen was injected intradermally into the volar surface of the forearm of those surveyed. The diameter of wheal and/or erythema was measured 15 minutes after injection. According to Ishizaki (1964), wheals over 9 mm in diameter and/or erythema over 20 mm in diameter were decided to be positive responses.

Positive persons were tested further by a twofold dilution series of the antigen solution to measure the threshold value because the titer thus determined resembled the reagin titer (Ishizaki, 1970).

5. *Field survey of O. nosophora*

A field survey of snail inhabitation in ricefields and their surroundings was made in October 1965 and October 1966. Each rice estate was checked on a map as to whether *O. nosophora* was found or not. Rice estates possessed by each of the three family groups were also shown separately on the map.

RESULTS

1. *Analysis of family histories*

Incidence of cirrhosis with ascites in a family including parents and brothers of the householder was compared with that of the three family groups mentioned above. There was, however, no significant difference among them probably because of the presence of patient(s) suffering from cirrhosis with ascites in most of the families surveyed. Some wives in families surveyed had come from nonendemic areas and were considered to be victims exposed to infection by *S. japonicum* without any protection. Ten wives belonging to that category were found in the three groups as shown in Table 1.

Table 1.   Summary of Data Obtained by Inquiry and Examination

Groups	Family unit					No. of members	Wives from nonendemic areas		
	No.	Cirrhosis in history	Cattle	Bare-foot	Night-soil		No.	*Schisto*. eggs in feces	Positive for skin test
Highly infected	7	5	4	7	7	31	3	3	3
Moderately infected	4	2	4	4	4	18	2	0	1
Uninfected	6	4	3	6	6	20	5	0	1
Total	17	11	11	17	17	69	10	3	5

Three wives in the highly infected group were of middle age (38, 46, and 58) at the time of the survey and all three stated that they had suffered from actute symptoms of schistosomiasis within a few months after their marriage. The symptoms were diagnosed as schistosomiasis and treated with Stibnal (sodium antimony tartarate). All three were found still positive for the skin test by schistosome antigen and showed schistosome eggs in their feces.

On the other hand, five wives in the uninfected group were all negative for schistosome eggs. Four of those had no experience of schistosomiasis and were negative for the skin test even though they had been engaged in farming for over 10 years in this area. Only one of them had experienced acute symptoms simulating schistosomiasis 8 months after her marriage. She had been treated but was still postivie for the skin test by schistosome antigen.

Two wives in the moderately infected group were negative for schistosome eggs in their feces even though they had 10 years of experience in farming in the area. But one of them showed a positive skin reaction to schistosome antigen, although she had no memory of symptoms which would suggest schistosomiasis.

Consequently, the occurrence of disease resulting from exposure to schistosome infection may vary greatly with families.

No difference in farming habits (rearing cattle and going barefoot) or use of nightsoil in their rice estates was observed among the three groups.

2. *Results of fecal examination and skin test*

Fecal examination: Results of the fecal examination and skin test by schistosome antigen are presented in Table 2. The egg-positive rate in the highly infected group is about three times higher than that in the moderately infected group. This fact may suggest that there are an average of 3 egg-positive cases in a family belonging to the highly infected group.

Table 2. Results of Fecal Examination and Skin Test

Groups	No. of members	Eggs (+) No. (%)	Skin test (+) by *S. japonicum* antigen (%) No.	Threshold value of skin test (grade diluted) Range	$\bar{x}$
Highly infected	31	20 (64)	25 (81)	8~4000×	580×
Moderately infected	18	4 (22)	13 (72)	4~ 500×	61×
Uninfected	20	0 (0)	10 (50)	8~ 130×	30×
Total	69	24 35	48 69		

The skin test-positive rates in the two infected groups were similar and the rate in the uninfected group was somewhat low. But the difference in the rates was not significant between the infected and uninfected groups. However, as already shown in Table 1, the skin test-positive rates in wives coming from nonendemic areas were significantly different among the three groups.

Threshold value (titer) of positive skin reaction: The threshold values in individuals surveyed are shown in Table 2 and Fig. 1 where abscissa and ordinate indicate age of individuals and their threshold values respectively. The values (represented in grade dilution) were high in the highly infected group and low in other two groups irrespective of age and presence of schistosome eggs in their feces.

From the facts that reagin production increased in individuals who were infected with the parasite and repeatedly stimulated with antigen and the threshold titer by skin test closely resembles the reagin titer in cases of schistosomiasis (Ishizaki, 1970), it would appear that infection in the highly infected group showing high threshold values in the skin test has occured more actively and recently than those in the other two groups.

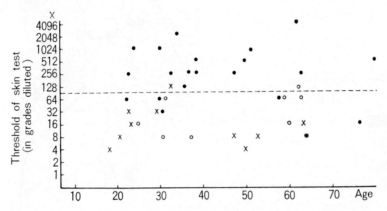

Fig. 1.   Correlation Chart of Threshold Values of Skin Test by Schistosome Antigen and Age Difference Among Three Groups.
●—Person in family of high infection
×—Person in family of moderate infection
○—Person in family of no infection

3. *Relation of geographical distribution of snails and rice estates owned by all three groups.*

The distribution of *O. nosophora* in the area is shown in Fig. 2 in which the estates owned by each of the three groups are also indicated, using a separate graphic pattern for each group. Careful inspection of the map shows that snails appeared to be distributed in estates along the central main irrigation canal running from north to south and that the estates owned by the highly infected group were located mainly where the snail was found. Those estates owned by the other two groups are located farther from the main canals and from the sites where the snail was found. From these observations it is concluded that human schistosome infection probably occurs mainly in small scattered places as small as a rice estate found in this area.

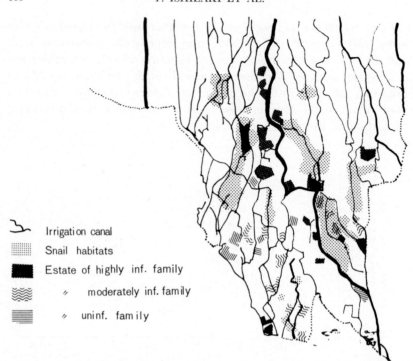

Irrigation canal
Snail habitats
Estate of highly inf. family
   ʺ   moderately inf. family
   ʺ   uninf. family

Fig. 2.   Relation of Geographical Distribution of Snail Habitats to Rice Estates
of the Three Groups Examined for Schistosomiasis Infection.

DISCUSSION

Though schistosomiasis japonica is still found in Japan, its endemic area has become smaller and the infection has tended to decrease in intensity during recent decades. Schistosome infection is, therefore, rarely found among those of the younger generation (Ishizaki, 1964). However, there are villages in some endemic areas where new infection continues to occur. The area surveyed is one of such endemic foci of schistosomiasis. The present investigation was carried out to ascertain where the infection occurs in relation to the intermediate host snails.

Family histories indicate that the endemic area was more highly contaminated by the parasite in the past. Most families surveyed had a record of one or more cases of cirrhosis with ascites, or death from it. A rather high positive rate of skin test in the three groups may be indicative of the previously wide occurrence of the infection.

It is an interesting and valuable fact that wives coming from nonendemic areas in each of the three groups reacted differently to the schistosome infection. Three wives in the highly infected group were infected with the parasite just after their marriage while 5 of 7 wives in the other two groups remained uninfected (no symptoms and negative skin test). This fact may suggest smaller foci where human infection occurs and a smaller number of snail habitats in the area.

As shown in Fig. 2, the distribution of threshold values (presented in grade dilution) shifted to the upper side in the cases of the highly infected group more than in those of the other two groups. That seems to be due to existing infection in the highly infected group and to infrequent or no occurrence in the other two groups.

Finally, the rice estates of families belonging to the highly infected group were inside the areas where the snail was found. But those of the other two groups did not always correspond to the snail habitats. The above mentioned facts in conjunction with common use of nightsoil in the rice fields in the area led to the conclusion that there is a close correlation between the occurrence of the infection and distribution of intermediate snails. The endemic foci of human schistosome infection are at present limited to small sites such as the rice fields owned by families in this area.

SUMMARY

An epidemiological survey was carried out to ascertain the foci of occurrence of schistosome infection in an endemic area in Yamanashi Prefecture, Japan.

Seventeen families containing 69 persons were divided into 3 groups: highly infected, moderately infected and uninfected family groups. Fecal examinations and skin tests with *S. japonicum* antigen were undertaken among all of them. Family histories and farming habits also served as tools in the present study. The snail survey was carried out in the rice estates of the endemic area in October 1965 and October 1966.

Results obtained are summarized as follows: Schistosomiasis in the area surveyed prevailed widely in the past and has decreased markedly in recent years. The foci where actual human infection by schistosome occurs are sites as small as rice estates owned by farming families in the area. The life cycle of *S. japonicum* may be maintained by a family (or domestic animal) as final host and by the intermediate host snails inhabiting the rice fields owned and simultaneously contaminated by the family.

REFERENCES

Ishizaki, T. (1964). A new criterion for the positive intradermal reaction to the antigen of *Schistosoma japonicum*. *Am. J. Trop. Med. & Hyg.*, **13**(5), 674.

Ishizaki, T. (1970). Skin tests in filariasis and schistosomiasis. Recent Advances in Research on Filariasis and Schistosomiasis in Japan, 331–353. Univ. Tokyo Press.

Melcher, L. R. (1943). An antigenic analysis of *Trichinella spiralis*. *J. Infect. Dis.*, **73**, 31.

Okabe, K. (1938a). The habitats of *Oncomelania nosophora* and the infection rate of *Schistosoma japonicum* in the Kofu Basin, Yamanashi Pref. *Kyudai Iho*, **12**(1), 23 (in Japanese).

Okabe, K. (1938b). The habitats of *O. nosophora* and the infection rate of *S. japonicum* in Fukuoka and Saga Pref., *Ibid.*, **12**(1), 28 (in Japanese).

Okabe, K. (1939). The habitats of *O. nosophora* and the infection rate of *S. japonicum* in Katayama district, Hiroshima Pref. *Ibid.*, **13**(3), 210 (in Japanese).

Ota S. and Sato S. (1957). Studies on several techniques for detecting the eggs of human parasite. *J. Kitakanto Igaku*, **7**, 68.

Studies on the Resistance of *Oncomelania* Snails to Molluscicides

K. YASURAOKA

Department of Parasitology, National Institute of Health,
Tokyo, Japan

INTRODUCTION

It is evident that complete eradication of the molluscan intermediate hosts would effectively put an end to the transmission of
schistosomiasis in any given area. The application of molluscicides is
considered at the present time to be the most promising and practical
single method in the control of schistosomiasis. Successful snail
control by means of molluscicides has been shown to be possible in
certain areas in Japan. Recently, Yurimin (3,5-dibromo-4-hydroxy-
4-nitroazobenzene), a new molluscicide developed in Japan, has
begun to compete with sodium pentachlorophenate (NaPCP) as a
molluscicide for routine snail control programs in Japan. However,
NaPCP is still one of the most commonly used molluscicides in this
country and almost all the endemic areas have been treated with this
compound twice a year, in spring and autumn when irrigation is not
in progress, since 1953. The amount of NaPCP sprayed so far in the
Yamanashi area is estimated to reach upward of 360 tons. The problem of resistance of *Oncomelania* snails to the molluscicide, whether
molluscicide-resistance develops in the repeatedly treated snail populations, has long been an interesting question for snail control programs in the prevention of schistosomiasis. There exist at present two
different and opposing views on development of resistance of snails
to molluscicides, one claiming such resistance (Okabe *et al.*, 1956;
Ota and Sato, 1956) and the other arguing against it (Walton *et al.*,
1958; Gancarz, 1958; Komiya *et al.*, 1961a, b; Yasuraoka *et al.*,
1971). The present paper briefly reviews and comments on the work
that has been done on the development of resistance of *Oncomelania*
to molluscicides.

SUMMARY OF PREVIOUS WORK

In 1956 Okabe *et al.* first called attention to the development of PCP-resistance in *Oncomelania nosophora* from the area treated with NaPCP. Using both plate and immersion methods, they compared the LC_{50} of snails collected in areas that had been treated with NaPCP for several years with that of snails obtained from untreated areas. The data in Table 1 indicate that the LC_{50} of the snails obtained from treated areas was higher than that of snails from untreated areas. It was concluded that a marked resistance to NaPCP had developed in areas where this molluscicide had been used for several years.

Table 1.   Resistance of *Oncomelania nosophora* to Sodium Pentachlorophenate (Okabe *et al.*, 1956)

Place	Test method	LD_{50}	Area
Nagatoishi	Plate	1 : 67 450	Treated
(Fukuoka Pref.)	Immersion	1 : 10 400	area
Ihara	Plate	1 : 157 000	
(Okayama Pref.)	Immersion	1 : 223 640	Untreated
Amagi	Plate	1 : 224 000	area
(Fukuoka Pref.)	Immersion	1 : 43 900	

At the same time Ota and Sato (1956) were studying the development of resistance to molluscicides. In this case the snails used were divided into two groups. One group was exposed from 1 to 6 hours to a solution containing 1:100 000 NaPCP. The survivors from this group were then exposed successively, at intervals of 1 week, to solutions containing 1:90 000, 1:80 000, 1:70 000, 1:60 000, 1:50 000, 1:40 000, 1:30 000, 1:20 000, and 1:10 000 of the compound. Corresponding numbers of snails from the control group were exposed to the same concentrations and the mortality of the two groups was compared. A similar test was made with dinitro-o-cyclohexylphenol (DN-1). The data from these experiments showed that the difference in the survival rates in the two groups of snails became more marked as exposure advanced. It was concluded from these results that resistance to these two molluscicides developed in *O. nosophora* after repeated exposure to increasing concentrations of the compounds.

Gancarz (1958) studied the development of resistance of *O. hupensis* to NaPCP, using a method similar to that of Ota and Sato

(1959). In this case the snails were exposed at intervals of 2 weeks, 1 month or 4 months to solutions containing predetermined concentrations equal to LC_{30}, LC_{50}, LC_{70} and LC_{90}. Altogether more than 14,000 snails were used. He found that the mortality rate of the experimental group was only slightly lower than that of the control group. It was concluded that the slight difference could not be attributed to the development of resistance.

Walton *et al.* (1958) conducted experiments similar to those of Okabe *et al.* (1956). An immersion test was used to compare the mortality rates of snails collected from areas that had been treated for several years with NaPCP and DN-1 with the rates of snails collected in nearby areas where the molluscicides had not been used. The results from these experiments are shown in Tables 2 and 3. The data in Table 2 show that resistance to NaPCP did not develop in snails from areas where this molluscicide had been used for 4 and 7 years. In Table 3, however, the data show that marked resistance to DN-1 developed in areas where this compound had been used for 6 years.

Komiya *et al.* (1961), using an immersion method, reexamined the development of resistance to NaPCP by comparing the LC_{50} of groups of snails collected in areas that had been treated with this

Table 2. Mortality of *O. nosophora* in Immersion Test with Sodium Pentachlorophenate (Walton *et al.*, 1958)

Immersion solution	Treated areas		Untreated areas		
	7 years	4 years	A	B	C
Tap water control	0/10	1/10	0/10	0/10	0/10
1.5 ppm NaPCP					
1	3/10	2/10	2/10	1/10	3/10
2	3/10	5/10	5/10	2/10	5/10
3	4/10	3/10	5/10	4/10	5/10
4	4/10	4/10	2/10	5/10	2/10
5	3/10	3/10	3/10	3/10	4/10
6	5/10	4/10	4/10	1/10	5/10
7	2/10	3/10	2/10	4/10	3/10
8	1/10	2/10	2/10	4/10	2/10
9	3/10	4/10	6/10	1/10	2/10
10	2/10	2/10	2/10	1/10	3/10
Total	30	33	33	26	34
% mortality	30	33	33	26	34

Table 3. Mortality of *O. nosophora* in Immersion Test with DN-1
(Walton *et al.*, 1958)

Immersion solution	Treated area	Untreated areas	
	Tanooka	Kagaminakajo	Imasua
Tap water control	0/10	0/10	0/10
1.5 ppm DN-1			
1	1/10	3/10	4/10
2	0/10	4/10	8/10
3	0/10	2/10	4/10
4	0/10	6/10	4/10
5	0/10	3/10	5/10
6	0/10	1/10	2/10
7	0/10	4/10	6/10
8	1/10	5/10	7/10
9	1/10	5/10	6/10
Total	3	31	46
% mortality	3.3	34.5	51.1

compound for 4 years with that of snails from untreated areas. The
results obtained are summarized below and indicate that the development of resistance to NaPCP was slight in these snails: the statistical
analysis of the mortality curve suggested that there was no significant
difference between the two.

Snails from treated areas
A $LC_{50} = 0.30$ ppm
B $LC_{50} = 0.32$ ppm

Snails from untreated areas
C $LC_{50} = 0.23$ ppm
D $LC_{50} = 0.25$ ppm

Komiya *et al.* (1961) studied further the various aspects of the
development of resistance. These included laboratory experiments
to determine: (a) the possible development of acquired resistance;
(b) the existence of resistant strains; and (c) if such strains exist, the
question whether they will develop greater resistance with higher
selection pressure.

In the first of these experiments snails were submerged in an
0.0625ppm solution of NaPCP for 48 hours (a sublethal exposure)
once every 3 weeks. A control group was submerged in water. After
three exposures of the experimental group, the LC_{50} of both groups
was determined and the results were as follows:

Experimental group — — — — — — $LC_{50} = 0.463$ppm
Control group — — — — — — — — $LC_{50} = 0.716$ppm

While the difference between these two groups was slight, the results indicated that exposure to small amounts of NaPCP under the conditions prevailing in this experiment might make the snails more susceptible.

In the second experiment the snails were exposed to predetermined concentrations equal to LC_{50} and LC_{90}. The LC_{50} of the survivors was then compared with that of control snails. The results given below show no marked difference between the three groups:

Snails surviving LC_{50} $-----$ $LC_{50}=0.224$ ppm
Snails surviving LC_{90} $-----$ $LC_{50}=0.243$ ppm
Controls $-----------$ $LC_{50}=0.216$ ppm

The survivors of the above experiment were reared in the laboratory and they produced offspring. To obtain dosage-mortality figures, offspring with a shell length of more than 6.0 mm were submitted to different concentrations of NaPCP. The results were:

Offspring of snails selected with $LC_{50}--LC_{50}=0.23$ ppm
Offspring of snails selected with $LC_{90}--LC_{50}=0.22$ ppm
Offspring of control snails $------LC_{50}=0.26$ ppm

On the basis of these experiments, it was concluded that no resistance develops either with repeated exposure to NaPCP or with a higher selection pressure of the compound.

Yasuraoka *et al.* (1971) made a long survey over 13 years to determine if resistance to NaPCP developed in snails from areas that had been treated twice a year with this molluscicide. In this study the

Table 4. LC_{50} of NaPCP in *Oncomelania nosophora* Snails from Treated Area in Each Year from 1958 to 1970 (Yasuraoka *et al.*, 1971)

Year	Number of tests	Average LC_{50} in ppm	SE
1954	5	0.31	± 0.07
1958	3	0.32	± 0.13
1959	3	0.26	± 0.09
1960	2	0.34	± 0.04
1961	11	0.33	± 0.08
1962	8	0.33	± 0.04
1963	4	0.36	± 0.05
1964	2	0.31	± 0.07
1965	4	0.32	± 0.07
1966	4	0.33	± 0.09
1967	5	0.30	± 0.05
1968	7	0.37	± 0.11
1969	3	0 30	± 0.05
1970	2	0 33	± 0.12

snails were collected from a treated area in Yamanashi Prefecture at intervals of 1 to 6 months and the LC_{50} was determined. The average LC_{50} values calculated in each year are listed in Table 4 and are graphically illustrated in Fig. 1. There was no significant change in the LC_{50} values all through the period of observation, indicating that no resistance to NaPCP develops even in snails from areas treated with the molluscicide for 18 consecutive years.

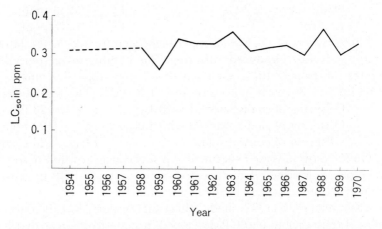

Fig. 1.   Change in LC_{50} of NaPCP in *Oncomelania nosophora* Snails from Treated Area in Each Year from 1958 to 1970. (Yasuraoka *et al.*, 1971).

COMMENTS

The above review shows that Okabe *et al.* (1956) and Ota and Sato (1956) believe that *Oncomelania* snails develop resistance to NaPCP, while the authors of the other publications (Walton *et al.*, 1958; Gancarz, 1958; Komiya *et al.*, 1961a, b; Yasuraoka *et al.*, 1971) have not confirmed these findings.

Both the immersion and plate techniques can be used for testing the susceptibility of amphibious *Oncomelania* snails to molluscicides. Okabe *et al.* (1956) used both plate and immersion techniques to compare the mortality rates of snails, while the other workers used only immersion techniques. The use of plate technique has been recommended by McMullen (1949) for the early evaluation of molluscicides against *Oncomelania* snails. This technique is of course the most satisfactory as a screening test, particularly for water-insoluble molluscicides, but it has some short-comings when used for water-soluble chemicals; this is because the snails come in contact with chemicals only with a part of their body, some snails move off the moist filter paper with the molluscicides, and at times some of them ingest a considerable amount of filter paper. All such activities appear to interfere with the accuracy and reproducibility of the effects.

The immersion technique would be superior to plate technique for comparative bioassay of the susceptibility of *Oncomelania* snails particularly to water-soluble chemicals because of its extreme accuracy and reproducibility. However, opinion was far from uniform among those who had worked with this technique concerning (1) the length of time during which snails are in contact with chemicals, (2) the temperature at which snails are in the solution, (3) the amount of the solution per snail during the test, and (4) the time of examining snails for their death. In addition, no step was taken to prevent snails from creeping out of the solution, with the exception of those in studies by Komiya et al. (1961) and Yasuraoka et al. (1971). Such a lack of uniformity does not guarantee a common basis for the comparison of data obtained in various laboratories. Efforts for the standardization of molluscicidal testing methods were pursued by Komiya et al. (1962) to ensure reproducibility and comparability of data obtained in various laboratories. The effect of factors upon the bioassay of molluscicides for *Oncomelania* snails was thoroughly studied, as a result of which a standardized immersion technique was established. Komiya, et al. (1961) and Yasuraoka et al. (1971), studying the resistance problem with this standardized technique, came to the conclusion that no resistance to NaPCP develops in *O. nosophora*. The difference between these results and those obtained by Okabe et al. (1956) and Ota and Sato (1956) may partially be ascribed to a lack of uniformity in immersion techniques used.

It has been pointed out by Tsuda (1952) and Yasuraoka, et al. (1966) that the susceptibility of snails to molluscicides varies with the season of the year. Much care should be exercised to avoid such seasonal variations in the comparative bioassay of the susceptibility of snails to molluscicides. Okabe et al. (1956) used snails collected from treated and untreated areas at different times of the year. For this reason, the data shown in Table 1 were selected so that they show only the results obtained from snails collected at the same time (6 June, 1956). Even with the elimination of the seasonal variable, the LC_{50} of the snails from the treated area is higher than that of snails from the untreated area. There is still the possibility that the rather widely separated geographical locations of the snail colonies have affected the results. In the experiments made by Walton, *et al.* (1958), Komiya *et al.* (1961) and Yasuraoka *et al.* (1971), the snails were collected from almost the same habitat in order to eliminate the possible geographical variable.

In the works reviewed herein, with the exception of that by Yasuraoka *et al.* (1971), the change of LC_{50} of snails was observed in a relatively short period of time, i.e. for only several generations of snails. Yasuraoka *et al.* (1971) conducted standardized immersion tests at intervals of 1 to 6 months for 13 consecutive years with snails from areas treated with NaPCP for as long as 18 years, which might involve at least 20 to 30 generations of snails. As a result, no significant change in the LC_{50} values was seen all through the period of observation. These data and the fact that in the practical use of NaPCP in the Yamanashi area at a dosage of 5 g/m² a satisfactory kill, 70–90% mortality, has been obtained ever since 1958 (Yasuraoka, 1970), support the view that no resistance develops with repeated applications of NaPCP.

Ota and Sato (1956) and Walton *et al.* (1958) have reported that *Oncomelania* snails develop resistance to DN-1. At this time it appears, however, that definite conclusions cannot be made on the development of resistance to DN-1 by *Oncomelania*. A fully satisfactory explanation of this problem can be advanced only after much more work has been done. For the moment it can be said with certainty that there is not any evidence that *Oncomelania* snails have acquired resistance to NaPCP.

However, it is necessary to be alert to this possibility. Investigations on this problem should include such aquatic snail hosts of schistosomes as *Biomphalaria* and *Bulinus* as well as *Oncomelania*.

REFERENCES

Gancarz, Z. (1958). Studies on schistosomiasis III. Resistance of *Oncomelania* snails to sodium pentachlorophenate. *Chinese Med. J.*, **77**, 236.

Komiya, Y., Yasuraoka, K., Hosaka, Y. and Ogawa, K. (1961). The resistance of the *Oncomelania* snail to molluscicides 1. Sodium pentachlorophenate. *Jap. J. Med. Sci. Biol.*, **14**, 131.

Komiya, Y., Yasuraoka, K. and Hosaka, Y. (1961). Review of studies on the resistance of *Oncomelania* snails to molluscicides in Japan. *Bull. Wld Hlth Org.*, **25**, 724.

Komiya, Y., Hosaka, Y. and Yasuraoka, K. (1962). Study for the standardization of quantitative test of the susceptibility of *Oncomelania* snails to sodium pentachlorophenate. *Jap. J. Med. Sci. Biol.*, **15**, 41.

McMullen, D. B. (1949). A plate method of screening chemicals as molluscicides. *J. Parasit.*, **35**, 28 (Suppl.).

Okabe, K., Okahara, T. and Ono, N. (1956). PCP-Na resistance of *Oncomelania nosophora* (Robson). *J. Kurume Med. Assoc.*, **19**, 1609. (text in Japanese with English summary).

Ota, S. and Sato, S. (1956). Resistance of *Oncomelania nosophora* to molluscicides. *Kitakanto Med. J.*, **6**, 287 (text in Japanese).

Tsuda, E. (1953). The relationship of the chemical resistance of *Oncomelania nosophora* to the seasonal period. *Tokyo Med. J.*, **69**, 48 (text in Japanese).

Walton, B. C., Winn, M. M. and Williams, J. E. (1958). Development of resistance to molluscicides in *Oncomelania nosophora*. *Amer. J. Trop. Med. & Hyg.*, **7**, 618.

Yasuraoka, K., Hosaka, Y. and Komiya, Y. (1966). Seasonal variation in the susceptibility of *Oncomelania nosophora* to sodium pentachlorophenate in relation to bioassay of molluscicides. *Jap. J. Med. Sci. Biol.*, **19**, 105.

Yasuraoka, K. (1970). Some recent research on the biology and control of *Oncomelania* snails in Japan. Recent Advances on Filariasis and Schistosomiasis in Japan. 291–303. Univ. Tokyo Press & Univ. Park Press.

Yasuraoka, K. and Hosaka, Y. (1971). Resistance of *Oncomelania* snails to sodium pentachlorophenate. *Jap. J. Med. Sci. Biol.*, **24**, 393.

Pathology of Liver Cirrhosis Due to
Schistosoma japonicum

H. Tsutsumi and T. Nakashima

*First Department of Pathology, Kurume University School of Medicine,
Kurume, Japan*

INTRODUCTION

The basin of the River Chikugo, near Kurume, is still one of the prominent areas in Japan whose population is infected with schistosomiasis japonica. Autopsies and biopsies done in this district often reveal schistosome eggs in the tissue specimens of each organ. In particular, the liver is almost always involved in schistosomiasis japonica either as a mild granulomatous lesion or as severe fibrosis. Very high pathological changes in the liver advancing to a stage of liver cirrhosis with schistosome eggs can be detected. The principal activities of Kurume University School of Medicine's department of pathology were comprehensive pathomorphological studies of liver cirrhosis due to *Schistosoma japonicum* carried out on autopsied and biopsied cases in humans and experimental cases in rabbits.

MORBIDITY OF SCHISTOSOMIASIS JAPONICA AT THE BASIN OF THE RIVER CHIKUGO

1. Autopsied cases.

Out of 2,263 cases which had been autopsied in this department from 1955 to 1968, the morbidity of the disease was 5.7% of all cases and 15.0% in cases of the epidemic area. In order to compare this morbidity rate with previous ones, the results of our predecessors' studies are given in Table 1.

2. Biopsied cases.

Histological observation was made on 770 surgical liver biopsied specimens which had been obtained by raparotomy between 1956 and 1960. The percentage of the egg positivity was 13.1% and was very high (53.9%) in cases of the endemic area, while that in 1,584 needle-biopsied specimens of the liver taken from 1950 to 1969 ac-

Table 1.   Morbidity in Human Autopsied Cases.

Reporter	Morbidity in all autopsied cases	Morbidity in autopsied cases at endemic area
Aonuma (1942)	13.9%	43%
Tanaka (1955)	15.3%	36.3%
Watanabe (1966)	4.7%	17.8%
Tsutsumi et. al. (1967)	5.7%	15.0%

counted for 7.7%. Yoshizumi (1955) reported that the egg was found by the fresh liver slide method in 60.1% of 113 cases from the endemic area whose inhabitants complained of various clinical symptoms.
3. Removed appendices.

The materials used in this study were collected from medical institutes in the area of Kurume and Tosu cities. In histological examination of 328 removed appendices by Tsutsumi et al. (1967), the percentage of the egg positivity was 7.6% and 12.1% in cases from the endemic area. Examination of 1,543 removed appendices using the histolysis method of Tobaru et al. (1969), revealed that it was 7.7% and 16.8% in cases from the endemic area. Results of previous studies are shown in Table 2 for comparison.

The morbidity of schistosomiasis japonica at the basin of the River Chikugo has recently decreased compared with its previous morbidity. With regard to annual morbidity from 1955 to 1968 (Fig. 1), no remarkable change in rate could be seen in autopsied cases. However, a small decrease was recognized in needle-biopsied cases after 1965.

Table 2.   Morbidity in Removed Appendices.

Reporter	Morbidity in all removed appendices
Komori (1938)	7.1%
Sagara (1941)	6.3%
Sagara (1948)	8.1%
Konishi (1966)	9.04%
Tsutsumi (1967)	7.6%
Tobaru (1969)	7.7%
	Morbidity in cases of the endemic area
Hashimoto (1951)	30.2%
Yoshioka (1954)	33%
Tsutsumi (1967)	12.1%
Tobaru (1969)	16.8%

HISTORICAL FINDINGS OF LIVER LESIONS IN SCHISTOSOMIASIS JAPONICA

The adult worm is parasitic in the portal vein. Embolus formation due to eggs occurs in the liver and digestive tract. Lesions in the liver are specific fibrosis, namely egg nodules are seen in the Glisson's capsule and distinct proliferation of the connective tissue can be recognized along the portal vein.

1. Fibrosis.

Fibrosis due to schistosomiasis in the liver is histologically classified into three types as follows (Nakashima, 1969).

1) Pipe-stem fibrosis.

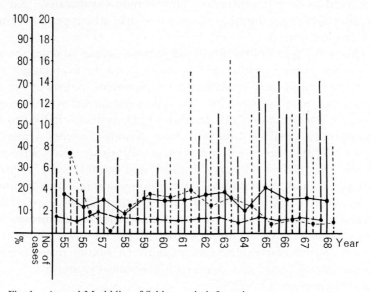

Fig. 1. Annual Morbidity of Schistosomiasis Japonica.
•, Percentage; - - - -, Needle-biopsied cases; ——, Cases in endemic area; —— Autopsied cases

Symmers (1904) noted a new form of liver cirrhosis due to the presence of the eggs of *Bilharzia haematobia* "The cut surface of the liver looked as if a number of white clay-pipe stems had been trust at various angles through the organ." The name "pipe-stem fibrosis" was used thereafter for specific liver cirrhosis due to *Schistosoma mansoni*. "Pipe-stem portal fibrosis," "periportal fibrosis," and "axial fibrosis" have also been used for the same form. Thus, pipe-stem fibrosis is one of the specific findings in liver lesions due to *Schistosoma japonicum*. It can be classified into two types:

i) Fiber zone with a hemangioma-like appearance. This fiber zone contains many dilated blood vessels and lymph vessels, presenting a hemangioma-like appearance. This finding depends mainly upon dilation of the vessel net around the bile duct and upon capillarization of the sinusoid after the disappearance of liver cells, and it plays the role of collateral circulation for circulatory insufficiency of the portal vein. ii) Fiber zone showing a whitish scar-like appearance. This fibrous tissue in the portal space consists of a dense whitish scar with poor vessels. This finding depends upon cicatrization after pylephlebitis and periphylephlebitis with the egg embolus and shows a marked hyaline degeneration. Destruction, calcification, and absorption of the eggs into this zone seem to take a long period of time.

   2) Septal fibrosis.

This is one type of liver fibrosis in schistosomiasis japonica. Septal formation causes a tortoise-shell appearance on the liver surface and connective tissue cord spreading from pipe-stem fibrosis in the cut surface can be recognized. This lesion does not spread over the whole liver, but it is circumscribed. Andrade (1965) believed that it was not necessary to separate this type from Symmers' type. However, Hashem (1947) described this type of fibrosis as "fine periportal fibrosis" or "diffuse bilharzial fibrosis" and Bogliolo (1957) agreed with this opinion. Septal fibrosis in schistosomiasis japonica is formed by connective tissue cords mutually connecting the interlobular Glisson's capsules as well as by connective tissue cord connecting the central vein and the Glisson's capsule. This finding is thought to show formation of collateral vessels against circulation disturbance of the peripheral portal vein due to schistosomiasis japonica.

   3) Postnecrotic fibrosis.

This fibrosis is mainly seen near the liver surface in severe schistosomiasis japonica. A few interlobular Glisson's capsules containing many egg nodules are seen in the same connective tissue. Transition patterns suggestive of degeneration, atrophy, necrosis, and disappearance of liver cells, close adherence of reticular fibers, and collagen formation can be seen. Andrade *et al.* (1961) reported that this localized postnecrotic fibrosis may have been induced by repeated ischemic insults tolerated for a long time, and by "piecemeal necrosis," possibly an expression of a chronic immunologic response. Although the author could recognize no immunological response by the fluorescent antibody technique in experimental liver fibrosis of rabbits, results agreeing with the "ischemic insult theory" could be obtained by a casting pattern of blood vessels in the liver.

2. Lesions of the portal vein.

As mentioned above, fibrosis in the portal space is conspicuous and of prime importance for the production of liver fibrosis in schistosomiasis japonica. Furthermore, intensive narrowing of the lumen, hyperplasia of the muscle layer, and a marked increase of elastic fibers followed by intimal fibrous thickening are also seen. These changes mean that the circulation disturbance has been a prolonged one. Portal inflammation has been described by practically every investigator of schistosomiasis, but intensive changes in the portal vein were reported by Fujinami (1916) in schistosomiasis japonica and by Lichtenberg (1955) in schistosomiasis mansoni.

3. Lesions of the hepatic artery.

Arterial lesions are not a pronounced feature in light and mild cases, but intimal fibrous thickening can be observed in most cases of severe schistosomiasis japonica. Andrade (1965) reported that "the arterioles present variable intimal fibrous thickening with narrowing of the lumens, which is basically a nonspecific reactive arteriolosclerosis probably produced by periarteriolar inflammation." We observed the hepatic arteries in experimentally infected rabbits showing conspicuous dilated and compensated portal circulation disturbance. It may be considered possible that arteriolosclerosis naturally occurs by continuous hypertension of the hepatic artery due to repeated infections.

4. Lesions of the bile duct.

In the majority of our autopsied cases, ductular proliferation and marked fibrosis around the bile duct were observed and the worms or eggs of *Clonorchis sinensis* were histologically detected in some cases. When these lesions are pronounced in the liver specimen, the presence of the complication of *Clonorchis sinensis* seems to be demonstrated by the fact that the basin of the River Chikugo has been well known as an endemic area of both schistosomiasis japonica and clonorchiasis. Andrade (1965) described focal bile ductal or ductular proliferation and periportal fibrosis in schistosomiasis mansoni. Fujinami (1916) reported that hyperplasia of the bile ductulus accompanying hyperplasia of the interstitium could be also observed in schistosomiasis japonica. In our experimental schistosomiasis japonica in rabbits, formation of pseudobile ductules and proliferation of bile ductules were occasionally observed.

CLASSIFICATION OF LIVER LESIONS
DUE TO *S. JAPONICUM*

Liver lesions due to *S. japonicum* are divided into first grade fibrosis, second grade fibrosis (liver fibrosis), and third grade fibrosis (liver cirrhosis). Cases which involved another type of liver cirrhosis are outside this classification. Table 3 shows the criteria of the classification.

Table 3. Classification of Liver Lesions Due to *S. japonicum*

	Gross findings	Histological findings
1st grade	Surface: smooth.	Egg emboli in peripheral Glisson's capsules alone.
2nd grade	Surface: shallow depressions. Cut surface: fibrosis.	Circumscribed fibrosis in middle-sized Glisson's capsules containing eggs as well as in peripheral capsules.
3rd grade	Surface: tortoise-shell appearance. Cut surface: pipe-stem fibrosis and septal fibrosis.	Septal fibrosis dividing liver parenchyma. Fiber zone containing egg nodules. Disorderly interdigitation between each intrahepatic vessel.

1. First grade fibrosis.

Cases in this category involve eggs contained in the peripheral Glisson's capsule alone and liver fibrosis is seldom seen. Macroscopically, the liver surface is smooth and eggs of *S. japonicum* can be recognized only through histological examination.

2. Second grade fibrosis (liver fibrosis due to *S. japonicum*)

Eggs are present in the middle-sized Glisson's capsule as well as in the peripheral Glisson's capsule. Septal formation due to proliferation of the connective tissues containing eggs can be seen. A great number of eggs are clustered limitedly below the capsule and the capsule shows a circumscribed thickening due to the fibrosis following the disappearance of the liver parenchyma at this site. The liver surface shows a shallow depression of the region mentioned above. Clinically, most cases in this grade are not diagnosed as s. japonica.

3. Third grade fibrosis (liver cirrhosis due to *S. japonicum*)

A tortoise-shell appearance on the liver surface due to thickening and a shallow or deep depression is extremely characteristic of this type. The liver in long-standing cases shows atrophy and its edge is rounded. Furthermore, the size of the right lobe is sometimes almost the same as the left lobe. Pipe-stem fibrosis and septal fibrosis are predominant in the cut surface of the liver. Many eggs are clustered, especially in the region of postnecrotic fibrosis. The frequency of liver cirrhosis due to *S. japonicum* was: Twenty-two cases of liver cirrhosis due to *S. japonicum* were seen among 152 cases of liver cirrhosis recognized by surgical biopsy during these 15 years (5.9%) and 20 cases of liver cirrhosis due to *S. japonicam* were seen among 229 cases of liver cirrhosis at autopsy (8.7%). Out of 153 autopsied cases of s. japonica, 20 cases of liver cirrhosis due to *S. japonicum* were seen (13.0%). Liver cirrhosis due to the present parasite was an unexpectedly rare occurrence.

EGG DISTRIBUTION IN ORGANS

S. hematobium, *S. mansoni*, and *S. japonicum* are all different, both as schistosoma parasitic in humans and in the egg distribution in the host. In schistosomiasis japonica, it is a well-known fact that the egg distribution varies with the host, with each strain of *S. japonicum*, and with the intensity of the infection. Distribution of *S. japonicum* eggs was examined in autopsied and experimental cases in our department. Materials examined were the intestines (stomach, duodenum, jejunum, ileum, cecum, appendix, ascending colon, transverse colon, descending colon, and sigmoid colon), liver, pancreas, lungs, kidneys, urinary bladder, spleen, and brain. Methods of examination were as follows:

Method I. Histolysis method by 30% KOH

A ten gram specimen of each tissue mentioned above was soaked in a 30% KOH solution and was dissolved in an incubator at 37°C for 12 hours. After complete dissolution of the tissue, the number of *S. japonicum* eggs was counted.

Method II. Histological method

Each intestine, 10cm in length, was rolled, cut routinely into paraffin sections, and stained with hematoxylin-eosin to examine the egg distribution in each layer of the intestines.

Method III. Transillumination method

The rectum mucosa in particular was examined by a transillumination method.

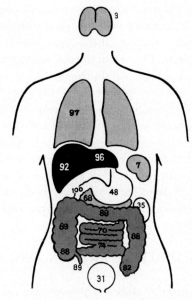

Fig. 2.   Egg Distribution in Cases of 1st and 2nd Grade Fibrosis.
The numeral at each organ indicates frequency of egg-positivity, and the density
of blackness indicates the relative number of eggs.

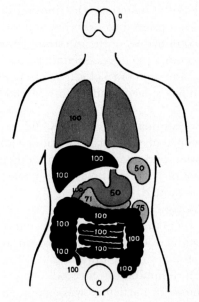

Fig. 3.   Egg Distribution in Cases of 3rd Grade Fibrosis (Liver Cirrhosis due to
S. *Japonicum*).
The numeral at each organ indicates frequency of egg-positivity, and the densi-
ty of blackness indicates the relative number of eggs.

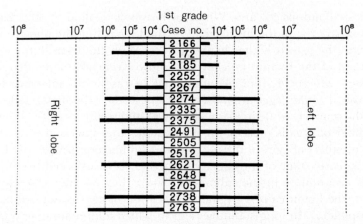

Fig. 4. Relationship between 1st Grade Fibrosis and Number of Eggs in the Liver.

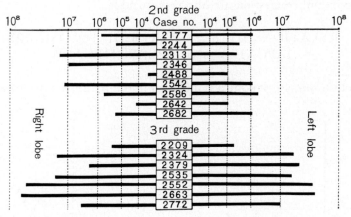

Fig. 5. Relationship between 2nd and 3rd Grade Fibrosis and Number of Eggs in the Liver.

The largest number of ova were seen in the liver, and the next largest in the digestive organs. They were scant in the spleen, kidneys, urinary bladder, and brain. In the digestive organs, ova were detected in the lower intestine more than in the upper and least in the stomach.

With regard to the grade of liver fibrosis, most ova are of the third grade showing intensive liver fibrosis, but the number of ova does not always run parallel with the grade of liver fibrosis.

Ova were usually present in the liver, digestive organs, and lungs in almost all autopsied cases. When the histolysis method by 30% KOH is compared with the histological method regarding the positive rate of ova, the rate is higher in the former. With the transillumination method of the rectum mucosa, ova show a remarkable tendency to cluster. Moreover, they are numerous in cases with intensive liver fibrosis. In man, eggs are most abundant in the submucosa, followed by the mucosa, while in the muscle layer and serosa a relatively small number of eggs is present. In the experimental infection in rabbits, the numbers of eggs in the mucosa and submucosa are equally large at the early stage of the egg-laying period. It is supposed that many eggs accumulate in the submucosa when they become obsolete. In man, the lesion caused by the intervention of eggs is not ordinarily conspicuous. In long-standing cases in which a large number of eggs exists, polyposis of the mucosa and thickness of the wall are recognized. In rabbits, the oval nodules are perceived through the serosa. Erosion and congestion are also recognizable.

RELATIONSHIP BETWEEN SCHISTOSOMIASIS JAPONICA AND SPLENOMEGALY

Schistosomiasis japonica is included in the Banti's syndrome and is

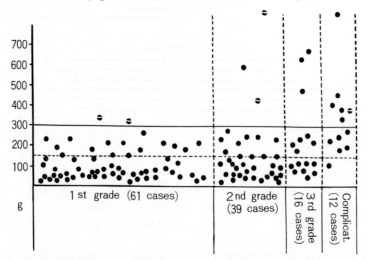

Fig. 6.   Spleen Weight in Autopsied Cases of Schistosomiasis Japonica. (128 Cases)

Complicat.: Cases which were complicated with liver cirrhosis of another type.
◒: Cases which involved reticulum cell sarcoma and myeloid leukemia.

known as one of the representative diseases with splenomegaly. Embolus formation of the portal vein, its organization, collapse of the peripheral branch, and thrombosis containing egg embolus are especially characteristic findings in schistosomiasis japonica. Although it seems clear that congestion causes splenomegaly, Fujinami (1965) considered that parasitism of *S. japonicum* also caused hyperplasia of the spleen directly or indirectly. It is often observed that splenomegaly does not always run parallel with the degree of hepatic lesion. Figure 6 shows the spleen weight in autopsied cases of schistosomiasis japonica.

Eggs are so rare in the spleen that the existence of eggs there is probably not closely related to splenomegaly. Comparison of the spleen weight in schistosomiasis japonica complicated with liver cirrhosis of other types with that in cases of liver cirrhosis due to schistosomiasis japonica alone disclosed that splenomegaly weighing over 300 g is more frequent in the former, and not as frequent as expected in the latter. Prata *et al.* (1963) reported that splenomegaly was rare even in advanced schistosomiasis mansoni. However, advanced splenomegaly is sometimes found in cases of schistosomiasis japonica, which is confirmed especially in surgery. The present author and associates should like to call cases with giant splenomegaly "a giant splenomegalic schistosomiasis japonica." On examination of the spleen weight and portal vein pressure in experimentally infected rabbits, the spleen weight gained with increase of portal vein pressure for 30 weeks after infection, and decreased with lowering of the portal vein pressure at the 40th week after infection. This stage in cases with a single infection corresponds to a term for recovery. In the light of experimental results obtained, it must be assumed that splenomegaly tends to recover with reconstruction of the liver.

RELATIONSHIP BETWEEN CANCER OF THE COLON AND LIVER, AND SCHISTOSOMIASIS JAPONICA

Consideration of the stimulation from parasites and the effects of eggs on the host leads us to presume that the parasite has some neoplastigenic factor. There is much literature on the relationship between schistosomiasis japonica and cancer of digestive organs. According to Kazama (1921), the frequency of cancer of the intestine was high in the endemic area of schistosomiasis japonica. Shimada

(1936) examined 13 cases of cancer of the colon, concluding that cancer easily arose in the rectum because of the egg stimulation produced by the high frequency of egg embolus there and because of other localized factors. Iuchi *et al.* (1970) studied the complication of liver cirrhosis and hepatoma in materials taken at biopsy, surgical biopsy, and autopsy and stated that 3 cases of hepatoma were confirmed in 42 cases of liver cirrhosis without schistosomiasis japonica (7.1%), while 19 cases of hepatoma were seen in 74 cases of liver cirrhosis with schistosomiasis japonica (25.7%).

Histologic and statistic examinations were made on 3,570 cases autopsied at Kurume University between 1929 and August, 1970. *S. japonicum* eggs were found in the liver of 190 cases of schistosomiasis japonica. Twenty-four cases of colon cancer and 3 cases of colon cancer with schistosomiasis japonica were recognized among all cases. Frequency of colon cancer with schistosomiasis japonica was $1.58 \pm 0.90\%$ and that of colon cancer without it $0.62 \pm 0.14\%$. Frequency of colon cancer in the former cases tended to be higher than in the latter. On histological examination of 12 cases of colon cancer with schistosomiasis japonica including 9 biopsied cases, there existed no distinct relationship between colon cancer and schistosomiasis japonica. However, only the relationship between the site of colon cancer and that of eggs could be suggested. Seventy-one cases of liver cancer were seen, of which 7 had schistosomiasis japonica. The frequency of liver cancer with schistosomiasis japonica was $3.68 \pm 1.37\%$ and that of liver cancer without it was $1.89 \pm 0.23\%$. The former was more frequent than the latter. All cases of liver cancer with schistosomiasis japonica mentioned above showed various degrees of lesions due to *S. japonicum*, but no positive findings in which the parasite concerned directly caused cancer could be obtained. Four cases of this affection proved to be atrophic liver cirrhosis. Although the relationship between liver cancer and schistosomiasis japonica was examined histologically and statistically, no distinct conclusion could be drawn even with a 90% confidence level in statistical observation, and no remarkable histological findings suggestive of it were obtained.

CONCLUSION

The basin of the River Chikugo is known as an endemic area of schistosomiasis japonica. Among the specimens obtained for biopsy and autopsy, lesions due to *Schistosoma japonicum* were frequently encountered. Morphological and statistical studies were carried out.

1) Morbidity of schistosomiasis japonica in the basin of the River Chikugo was 13.1% in surgical biopsied specimens of the liver, 7.6 to 7.7% in removed appendices, 7.7% in needle-biopsied specimens, and 5.7% in all autopsied cases. Morbidity of inhabitants in the endemic area of schistosomiasis japonica was 53.9% in surgical biopsied specimens, 12.1 to 16.8% in removed appendices, and 15.0% in autopsied cases. Change in annual morbidity from 1955 to 1968 was not remarkable in autopsied cases.

2) Examination of the egg distribution in each organ revealed that eggs were most frequent in the liver, their number diminishing in the following order: Sigmoid colon, cecum, descending colon, transverse colon, ascending colon, appendix, ileum, jejunum, duodenum, pancreas, lungs, stomach, urinary bladder, kidneys, spleen, and brain.

3) Although no remarkable difference between the number of eggs and the degree of liver fibrosis could be seen in first grade fibrosis or in second grade fibrosis (liver fibrosis), eggs were exceedingly numerous in third grade fibrosis (liver cirrhosis).

4) Although the adult worm in schistosomiasis japonica was not the direct pathogen of liver cirrhosis, its eggs were the main cause of the present disease. Complicated histological findings were obtained depending upon the differences in the developmental period of eggs and whether the eggs were laid in a highly sensitive or an immune period of the host.

5) Pipe-stem fibrosis, septal fibrosis, and postnecrotic fibrosis were encountered as liver fibrosis in schistosomiasis japonica.

6) A fiber band showing an angioma-like appearance and a fiber band showing a white cicatrified appearance were seen in pipe-stem fibrosis. The morphological development of pipe-stem fibrosis could not be definitively explained.

7) Diffuse septal and localized septal formation were seen in septal fibrosis. In the former, capillarization of the sinusoid could be seen in the septum except hyperplasia of the interlobular connective tissue. Maldistribution of eggs and adult worms in the liver might play a very important role in forming the localized septum.

8) Postnecrotic fibrosis was often seen in severe cases of infection. Intense circulation disturbance of the portal vein due to formation of emboli and egg nodules, narrowing of the collateral vein due to contraction of the connective tissues, and decompensation of the hepatic

artery due to thickening of the intima proved to be very important in inducing postnecrotic fibrosis.

9) Dilation of capillaries around the portal vein and capillary nets around the bile duct, seen in cases with portal circulation disturbances, led to recanalization of the embolized area in the portal vein, showing the presence of collateral circulation.

10) Sclerosis of the hepatic artery was often seen in cases of liver cirrhosis.

11) Nodular hyperplasia and formation of pseudobile duct in the liver parenchyma were not common in schistosomiasis japonica.

12) Liver lesions in schistosomiasis japonica were classified into three groups according to the grade of fibrosis. In first grade fibrosis, the liver surface was smooth and, histologically, the egg embolus was seen only in a small Glisson's capsule. Fibrosis was slight. In second grade fibrosis, a shallow depression on the liver surface was seen and septal formation was predominant in the cut surface. Histologically, eggs were found scattered also in middle-sized Glisson's capsules in the interlobular connective tissues, and below the capsule. Liver fibrosis was dominant. Third grade fibrosis corresponded to liver cirrhosis due to schistosomiasis japonica. The liver surface showed a lobular or a tortoise-shell appearance. Pipe-stem fibrosis, septal fibrosis, and postnecrotic fibrosis were seen in the cut surface. Histologically, besides eggs scattered below the capsule and in the septum, many egg nodules tended to gather in the site of postnecrotic fibrosis depending upon atrophy and disappearance of liver cells. Intense narrowing and thickening of the branches of the portal vein due to hyalization of emboli and egg nodules, as well as meandering of the branches of the portal vein due to liver atrophy, were seen.

13) Out of 152 cases of liver cirrhosis, 22 cases due to schistosomiasis japonica were seen in biopsied materials (5.9%). Out of 229 cases of liver cirrhosis, 20 cases due to *S. japonicum* were seen in autopsied cases (8.7%). Twenty cases of liver cirrhosis due to *S. japonicum* were found in 153 autopsied cases of schistosomiasis japonica (13%).

14) Although giant splenic schistosomiasis japonica was considered one of the Banti's syndromes, cases with the spleen weighing over 300g were small in number and the giant spleen was predominant in cases associated with other types of liver cirrhosis.

15) Marked egg accumulation in the rectum mucosa was generally seen in advanced fibrosis of the liver. Eggs tended to scatter in the rectum mucosa.

16) Colon and liver cancers with schistosomiasis japonica tended to be higher in frequency than cases without. Although the relationship between cancer of these organs and schistosmoiasis japonica was examined histologically and statistically, no distinct conclusion could be drawn even at the probability level of 90% in statistical examination and there were no remarkable histological findings suggesting that this relationship could be confirmed.

REFERENCES

Andrade, Z. A. (1965). Hepatic schistosomiasis, morphological aspects. Progress in liver disease II. Popper, H. and Schafner, F. Eds., 228, Grune & Stratton, New York and London.

Andrade, Z. A., Paronetto, F. and Popper, H. (1961). Immunocytochemical studies in schistosomiasis. Amer. J. Path., **39**, 589.

Bogliolo, L. (1957). The anatomical picture of the liver in hepato-splenic schistosomiasis mansoni. Ann. trop. Med. Parasit., **51**, 1.

Fujinami, K. (1916). [Pathological anatomy of schistosomiasis japonica.] Jap. J. med. Prog., **6**, 101.

Hanada, H., Kaneko, H., Tobaru, M., and Toyonaga, H. (1965). Statistical and pathological observations of schistosomiasis japonica based on 770 cases of liver biopsies, Part I: Statistical observations. J. Kurume med. Ass., **28**, 103.

Hashem, M. (1947). The etiology and pathogenesis of the endemic form of splenomegaly, the Egyptian splenomegaly. J. Roy. Egypt. med. Ass., **30**, 48.

Hasuda, A. (1967). Distribution of ova in the digestive tract in the cases of schistosomiasis japonica. J. Kurume med. Ass., **30**, 501.

Iuchi, M., Nakayama, Y., Ishiwa, M., Yamada, H., Chiwa, K., Iio, M., and Kameda, H. (1971). Studies on primary carcinoma of liver associated with schistosomiasis japonica. Intern. Med., **27**, 761.

Kazama, Y. (1921). [On the intestinal cancer in schistosomiasis japonica and on the etiological relationship between its genesis and the eggs.] Gann, **15**, 159.

Lichtenberg, F. (1955). Lesions of the intrahepatic portal radicles in Manson's schistosomiasis. Amer. J. Path., **31**, 757.

Nakashima, T. (1969). [Liver cirrhosis due to Schistosoma japonicum (I): Human cases.] Acta hepat. jap., **10**, 485.

Ninomiya, K. (1970). Studies on distribution of the ova of Schistosoma japonicum in organs with schistosomiasis japonica. J. Kurume med. Ass., **33**, 1375.

Prata, A. and Andrade, Z. A. (1963). Fibrose hepatica de Symmers sem esplenomegalia. Hospital (Rio de Janeiro), **63**, 617.

Shibata, T. (1968). Morphologic studies on chronic schistosomiasis japonica: Studies on complication of schistosomiasis japonica. J. Kurume med. Ass. **31**, 1237.

Shimada, H. (1936). [A case of rectostenosis in schistosomiasis japonica.] J. Chiba med. Soc., **14**, 294.

Symmers, W. (1904). Note on a new form of liver cirrhosis due to the presence of the ova of Bilharzia haematobia. J. Path. Bact., **9**, 237.

128   H. TSUTSUMI AND T. NAKASHIMA

Tobaru, M., Toyonaga, H., Akagi, T., and Kojima, T. (1966). Statistical and pathological observations of schistosomiasis japonica based on 770 cases of liver biopsies, Part II. Histological findings. *J. Kurume med. Ass.*, **29**, 945.

Tobaru, M , Ozasa, T , and Shibata, T (1969). Chronic schistosomiasis japonica and appendicitis. *J. Kurume med. Ass.*, **32**, 179.

Tsutsumi, H., Watanabe, A., and Nakashima, T. (1963). Studies on liver fibrosis (cirrhosis) due to schistosomiasis japonica: Morphology of liver, Part I. *Kurume med. J.*, **10**, 51.

Tsutsumi, H., Watanabe, A., and Nakashima, T. (1963). Studies on liver fibrosis (cirrhosis) due to schistosomiasis japonica: Morphology of liver, Part II. *Kurume med. J.*, **10**, 269.

Tsutsumi, H. and Hasuda, A. (1964). Studies on liver fibrosis (cirrhosis) due to schistosomiasis japonica: III. The state of intervention of ova in the digestive tract. *Kurume med. J.*, **11**, 80.

Tsutsumi, H., Ito, T., Ninomiya, F., and Kuwano, K. (1967). Schistosomiasis japonica and appendicitis. *J. Kurume med. Ass.*, **30**, 282.

Tsutsumi, H., Ozasa, T., Matsunaga, M., Ito, T., Ninomiya, F., and Ninomiya, K. (1971). Relationship between cancer of the colon and liver and schistosomiasis japonica. *J. Kurume med. Ass.*, **34**, 319.

Watanabe, A. (1966). The morphological studies on the liver cirrhosis due to schistosomiasis japonica. *J. Kurume med Ass.*, **29**, 772.

Yoshizumi, Y., Kuroda, I., Watanabe, H., and Oda, T. (1955). Further observations of schistosomiasis japonica by needle biopsy of the liver (Fresh liver slide method). *Kurume med. J.*, **2**, 63.

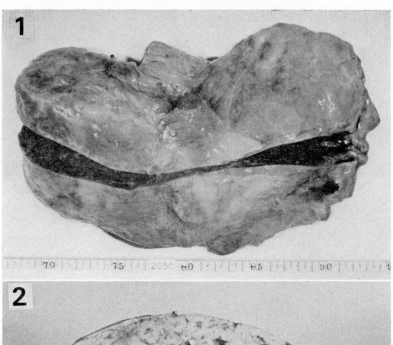

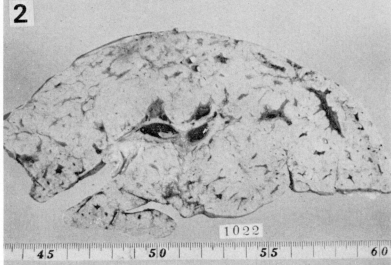

1. Surface of Liver Cirrhosis due to *S. japonicum*, No. 2050.

The tortoise-shell appearance on the liver surface due to thickening and a shallow or a deep depression is characteristic. This liver shows atrophy and its edge is rounded. Furthermore, the size of the right lobe is almost the same as the left.

2. Cut Surface of Liver Cirrhosis due to *S. japonicum*, No. 1022.

Pipe-stem fibrosis and septal fibrosis are predominant.

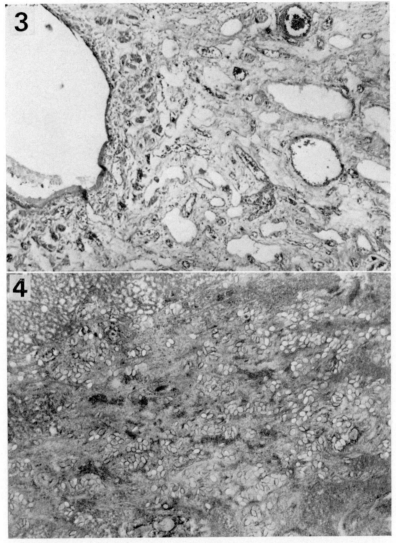

3. Fiber Zone Showing a Hemangioma-Like Appearance (Pipe-Stem Fibrosis) in Liver Cirrhosis due to *S. japonicum*, No. 2040. H. & E Stain. × 40. This fiber zone contains many dilated blood vessels and lymph vessels.

4. Fiber Zone Showing a Whitish Scar-Like Appearance (Pipe-Stem Fibrosis) in Liver Cirrhosis due to *S. Japonicum*, No. 1027. H. & E Stain. × 20.

This fiber zone consists of dense connective tissue containing many eggs and poor vessels.

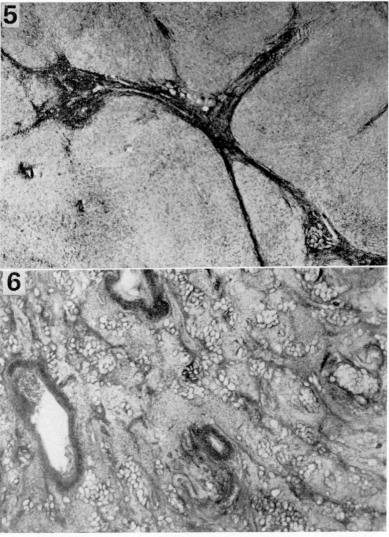

5. Septal Fibrosis in Liver Cirrhosis due to *S. japonicum*, No. 1022. Azan-Mallory Stain. × 20.

This type of fibrosis is formed by connective tissue cords mutually connecting the interlobular Glisson's capsules as well as by those connecting the central vein and Glisson's capsule.

6. Postnecrotic Fibrosis in Liver Cirrhosis due to *S. japonicum*, No. 1306. Azan-Mallory Stain. × 20.

A Few of the interlobular Glisson's capsules containing many egg nodules are seen in the same connective tissue.

Experimental Schistosomiasis Japonica in Rabbits

H. Tsutsumi and T. Nakashima

First Department of Pathology, Kurume University School of Medicine, Kurume, Japan

INTRODUCTION

When liver cirrhosis with schistosomiasis japonica is encountered at autopsy or biopsy, the parasite makes it very difficult to analyze the morphological development of liver cirrhosis. Exact pathological studies on this liver lesion cannot be carried out without first studying experimental schistosomiasis japonica. Seriously infected rabbits died in an acute stage of infection because of severe disturbance in the liver and digestive organs before the occurrence of liver cirrhosis in those organs. Therefore, it was necessary to control the number of cercariae in order to observe the morphological development of liver cirrhosis. Young male rabbits were used as experimental animals. Each rabbit received about 300 to 500 cercariae through cutaneous infection. Observations were carried out for 2 to 40 weeks thereafter.

MORPHOLOGICAL FINDINGS OF THE LIVER

Macro- and microscopic examinations were made at autopsy. Histological specimens were cut into serial sections, and stained by H & E and Azan-Mallory staining for stereographical scrutiny by the sketching reconstruction method.

1. *Process of development of liver cirrhosis due to* Schistosoma japonicum.
   1). Immature worms of *S. japonicum* first appeared within the branches of the intrahepatic vein 20 days after infection. Egg laying began 4 to 5 weeks after infection, and egg nodules were formed according to the maturation of egg contents. A sketch drawn by the reconstruction method of serial sections of the liver showed that lesions first occurred in the terminal twigs or in the axial distributing veins, and then extended to the surrounding liver parenchyma. Be-

[133]

fore the deposition of ova, no remarkable changes were found in the liver tissues except for dilatation of the portal branches.

2). Six weeks after infection, the egg embolism rapidly spread towards the proximal side of the portal vein, namely, from the terminal twig to the axial distributing and conducting veins. The leucocytic thrombus with matured eggs caused not only thrombopylephlebitis, peripylephlebitis, and portal hepatitis, but also the degeneration and disappearance of liver cells around those lesions. In the dilated sinusoid and inlet venules new exudative egg nodules were also seen. Pylephlebitis and portal hepatitis were the most significant factors of liver fibrosis due to *S. japonicum*.

3). The gross appearance of the liver, 8 weeks after infection, included a small number of white spots on the liver surface, but in 10 weeks the egg nodules increased in number, enlarged in size, and partially conglutinated with one another so that the connective tissue was seen proliferating around the oval nodules while neighboring nodules were also wrapped in the same connective tissue.

4). The liver surface, 18 to 20 weeks after infection, gave the appearance of an irregular tortoise-shell appearance, and showed conspicuous thicking of the capsule and dilatation of the superficial veins. Histologically portal phlebitis and periphlebitis were extensive, indicating advanced destruction, degeneration and disappearance of the liver parenchyma. The connective tissue interwove a mass of the liver parenchyma and a few liver cells. There was also the formation of a few new oval nodules among the liver parenchyma which maintained its lobular structure. Thus pipe-stem fibrosis or periportal fibrosis was formed.

5). Thirty weeks after infection, irregular indentations were conspicious all over the surface, giving a typical tortoise-shell appearance with flattening of coarse nodules. Histologically, numerous dilated small blood vessels were found within the fibrous band, and the borderline between the fibrous band and liver parenchyma was indistinct. At the portion of advanced fibrosis the limiting plate was clearly demarcated. In the parenchyma, some tendency towards nodular hypertrophy was observed and septal fibrosis surrounding the liver parenchyma appeared. In other sites, nodular hypertrophy of the liver parenchyma was definitely noted. Such a histological picture was similar in appearance to liver cirrhosis of type A or A'(Miyake) in the general classification of liver cirrhosis. In this stage, new oval nodules decreased in number.

Consequently, the morphology of the liver in experimental rabbits 20 to 30 weeks after infection might correspond to liver cirrhosis stemming from *S. japonicum.*

2. *The repairing process of the liver following the cirrhotic state.*

1). The beginning of the repairing process differs according to the degree of infection, the number of ova laid, spawning period, species of infected animals, and capacity for survival of the individual parasite. In our experiments, localized portal phlebitis or periphlebitis due to the ova embolism had already undergone repair by the 18th week. In liver cirrhosis due to *Schistosoma japonicum* fibrosis formed progressively and spread on the one hand, and repair took place simultaneously through proliferation of liver cells on the other, presenting various stages in both processes. Between 20 and 30 weeks after infection, morphology of the liver was maintained at the acme stage followed by a dominant process of repair.

2). Forty weeks after infection the liver showed a partially cicatricial depression with some flattening of the liver surface. Histologically, organization and recanalization were noted in the ovum emboli of the larger portal branches, giving a hemangioma-like appearance and resembling pipe-stem fibrosis of liver cirrhosis due to *S. japonicum* in man. Part of the septal fibrosis was loosened and liver cells arranged in a lamellar fashion appeared among the fiber bands. In addition, the loosened septal fibrosis assumed a fine appearance through proliferation of liver cells. Within the pipe-stem fibrosis, budding of liver cells was also noted.

CHANGES OF ANGIOARCHITECTURE
IN THE LIVER

Synthetic resins of colors which varied according to each blood vessel in the hepatic arterial, venous, and portal systems were injected to prepare casting patterns. In other livers, colored gelatin solution was given to apply the transillumination method.

1. About 10 weeks after infection the entrance of resin was inhabited in the peripheral branches of the portal system. There were collapse, deformity, and dilatation of their side branches. On the other hand, the peripheral arterial branches were dilated, elongated, and increased in number. The arterial system was intensely dilated, reaching a size several times larger than normal with a marked

tortuosity. The entrance of arterial capillaries into the oval nodules and the compensatory inflow of the arterial system into the peripheral sinusoid were observed.

2. The lumen of the peripheral portal vein 18 weeks after infection was almost occluded by pylephlebitis and peripylephlebitis containing egg emboli. Thrombosis further extended into the lumen of the larger proximal branches. Dilatation of the inlet venules and marginal sinusoid was conspicuous and new thrombus formation was noted in these lumina. Thus portal phlebitis and periportal inflammation around the egg embolus extended toward the proximal side of the liver, indicating progress into pipe-stem fibrosis.

3. Twenty weeks after infection, the tips of the portal branches were destroyed and their proximal side was intensely dilated. Numerous branches derived from this site forming a flower-like arrangement with irregular dilatation. Collapse, flattening and deformity of the portal vein, elongation and dilatation of the artery, development and dilatation of the peribiliary vascular net, and disorder of interdigitation between each vascular system were pronounced. In the portion with intense vascular changes smaller blood vessels with mixed color tones consisting of arterial and portal systems were present.

4. Thirty weeks after infection, dilatation of the arterial system, development of the peribiliary vascular network, shortening, engorgement, and deformity of the portal vessels remained, along with disorder of interdigitation between each vascular system. The course of arterial and portal system was regaining its balance.

5. Forty weeks after infection, development of the peribiliary vascular net, engorgement, deformity, and shortening of the portal vein partially remained. Most of the interdigitations in each vascular system were restored to normal. The specimens prepared after infusion of colored gelatin showed that the course of small blood vessels was almost normal.

LIVER FUNCTION TESTS

There are many reports on enzymatic studies of the serum in schistosomiasis. Nakano (1969) examined SGOT, SGPT, and Al-P in experimental rabbits with moderate infection.

1. *Changes of serum transaminase*
Nakano recognized the same sharp increase of SGOT and SGPT

in cases 4 weeks after infection as that reported by Sano (1960) and Kitajima (1967). In comparison with the histological findings, Nakano suspected that increase of transaminase depended upon transition of the intracellular enzyme to the blood flow following destruction of liver cells, mechanical stimulation of the egg, and increased permeability of the cell membrane due to metabolic and toxic substances of eggs. However, since recovery of transaminase to normal limits 8 weeks after infection did not fit into findings on the histological development of liver lesions, the increase of transaminase could not be explained satisfactorily.

2. *Changes of Al-P in the serum.*

Sano described the decrease of Al-P in the early stage of infection as ascribable to disturbance by egg toxin of Al-P production in the liver. He also considered that increase of Al-P 6 to 8 weeks after infection depended upon the obstruction of Al-P discharge by the inflammatory process of egg nodules. Nakano stated that the liver lesion in schistasomiasis was a circumscribed one, and that, however partial the disturbance of Al-P discharge might be, the liver could compensate through an active compensatory function. He therefore assumed that other factors participated in increase of Al-P.

3. *Changes of serum protein*

Changes in serum protein can be seen in liver disorders. It was suspected that the main cause for changes in serum protein might be its abnormal metabolism when serum protein production was disturbed. Interpretation of the increase of γ-globulin was not yet established. Various possible causes included the following: 1) extrahepatic production, 2) production by the plasma cell, 3) production by the reticuloendothelial system, 4) production by autoantibody, and 5) production by liver disorder.

Increases in total serum protein, decrease of albumin, and a sharp increase in globulin (especially γ-globulin) were demonstrated in schistosomiasis. Total serum protein increased to a marked degree 8 weeks after infection on the basis of the absolute increase of globulin (especially γ-globulin) in proportion to the decrease of albumin, while a slight increase of either α_1-gl. or α_2-gl. could be recognized 8 to 20 weeks after infection. The latter increase is thought to depend upon the exudative necrotic lesion, the subsequent tissue destruction, and the hyperplastic lesion. Definite increase of β-globulin is frequently cited in literature on experimental schistosomiasis. Furusawa (1958) stated that a relatively long-standing functional disorder of the protein metabolism was a distinct feature of schistosomiasis japonica confirmed in the liver function tests. Hirayama (1957) reported that β-globulin increased in many cases of the liver disease.

MORPHOLOGICAL DEVELOPMENT OF PIPE-STEM FIBROSIS

As a typical fiber band, Symmers' pipe-stem fibrosis and Hashem's diffuse bilharzial fibrosis could be seen in liver lesions due to schistosomiasis japonica as well as schistosomiasis mansoni.

1. *Pipe-stem fibrosis*

The histological pattern called pipe-stem fibrosis can be subdivided into: (1) periportal fibrosis with an angioma-like appearance and (2) periportal fibrosis with a white cicatrice appearance, which were both observed in autopsied cases. However, the cases examined of experimental schistosomiasis japonica of rabbits belonged mostly to the former type.

Relationship between pipe-stem fibrosis and eggs: with regard to the morphological development of pipe-stem fibrosis in the experiment on rabbits, mature eggs caused an intense thrombotic pylephlebitis in the terminal twigs as well as in the relatively large branches of the intrahepatic portal vein. Later, they were destroyed and disappeared. Therefore, only a few eggs were seen in long-standing fiber bands. Portal circulation disturbances and periportal fibrosis following thrombotic pylephlebitis and peripylephlebitis caused the destruction and disappearance of liver cells. Subsequently, accumulation of the gitterfasern and thickening of the connective tissues were seen, and a comparatively wide fibrosis was formed in that region as compared with the number of eggs.

The border of pipe-stem fibrosis and the liver parenchyma: though the limiting plate attaching to the exudative egg nodules was destroyed in the early stage of its nodule production, it was later formed anew by liver cells regenerating after the disappearance of inflammation. It was revealed that liver cells were regenerated in the bordering area between the fiber band and the liver parenchyma following reduction of pylephlebitis and peripylephlebitis occurring around the mature eggs as acute liver lesions. The border of the liver parenchyma and the fiber band then became more distinct.

The angioma-like appearance of pipe-stem fibrosis: The reconstruction method of serial sections of the liver led us to conclude that the angioma-like appearance of pipe-stem fibrosis is a result of intense dilatation of the portal vein, recanalization of the thrombus, dilatation of capillary nets around the bile duct as collateral circulation, and capillarization of the sinusoid due to the disappearance of liver cells.

2. *Septal fibrosis*

Septal fibrosis is different from pipe-stem fibrosis in the mechanism of development. Septal fibrosis is mainly represented by hyperplasia of the connective tissue and is formed by the connection of relatively small Glisson's capsules. Although some authors denied the significance of distinguishing between septal fibrosis and pipe-stem fibrosis, the former fibrosis is more pronounced in the reconstruction period of liver lesion due to schistosomiasis japonica in rabbits than in its developmental stage. Predominant septal fibrosis could be demonstrated 20 weeks after slight infection and 30 weeks after moderate infection; with the subsidence of peripylephlebitis a comparatively wide periportal fibrosis occurring in the process of development got loose and became disjointed in layers by regenerated liver cells, making the septum almost correspond to the course of the axial distributing vein and the conducting vein. This tendency became more conspicuous 40 weeks after infection through various stages of a marked, an interrupted, or a nearly reduced septum.

RECOVERY OF LIVER LESIONS

Though morphological studies on the development of liver cirrhosis due to schistosomes were carried out by many investigators, only a few reports have so far been made on the repairing process of the present disease. In liver cirrhosis due to worms, it was generally agreed that few hyperplastic nodules usually seen in portal or postnecrotic cirrhosis were formed. Andrade (1962) reported that passive or active nodules were present locally, and that they were only seen around the large Glisson's sheath and below the capsule. However, such hyperplastic nodules were detected in the liver parenchyma in certain stages of experimental liver lesions with schistosomiasis japonica as stated above. The presence of these nodules seemed to represent the repairing process of liver lesions. They were definitely distinguishable from the interstitium and the limiting plate was formed anew by the regenerated liver cell band running parallel with the interstitial connective tissues. The septum was loosened in layers from the margin of the acinus by the regenerated liver cell band, and the interstitium was also interrupted, divided, and thinned away by them. Experiments of schistosomiasis japonica in rabbits revealed that the liver cells supported by the remaining gitterfasern were regenerated in the interstitium in the course of recovery of liver lesions. Furthermore, it was found that the hyperplastic nodules were also formed at some stage of the disease as well as in general liver cirrhosis.

Accelerating factors in the regeneration of the liver cells are as follows:

1) marked decrease in egg laying, 2) contraction of egg nodules after healing of exudative inflammation, 3) formation of collateral circulation in damaged branches of the portal vein, and 4) disappearance of peripylephlebitis or others.

CONCLUSION

1. Liver lesions in schistosomiasis japonica in rabbits occurred first as an exudative necrotic lesion around the mature eggs embolized in the terminal twigs, and then spread to the proximal branches of the portal vein followed by thrombotic pylephlebitis and peripylephlebitis.

2. Most of the liver lesions in schistosomiasis in rabbits were caused directly or indirectly by eggs, especially by mature eggs.

3. Characteristic of the liver lesions occurring in schistosomiasis in rabbits were septal fibrosis and pipe-stem fibrosis with an angioma-like appearance.

4. The disturbance of intrahepatic portal circulation was very severe in liver lesions due to schistosomiasis. There were dilated capillary nets around the bile duct and egg nodules, compensating circulation disturbance in long-standing cases, while in the early stage there existed dilatation and elongation of the hepatic arteries as compensation.

5. In rabbits with a moderate infection of schistosomiasis, the

characteristic morphology of liver cirrhosis was found 20 to 30 weeks after infection, and reconstruction was recognized 30 weeks after in accordance with decreasing egg laying.

6. SGOT and sGPT were found to rise in value 4 weeks after infection, they fell 8 weeks after, and recovered to normal in 12 weeks. Serum Al-P decreased between 8 and 20 weeks after infection.

7. With regard to changes in serum protein, the A/G ratio decreased markedly 8 weeks after infection. Both the absolute and relative volumes of albumin also decreased in 8 weeks, whereas those of α-globulin increased in as many weeks. β-globulin increased 8 weeks after infection and recovered to normal after 20 weeks. γ-globulin increased in 8 weeks and gradually rose until the 20th week.

8. Experimental liver cirrhosis due to *S. japonicum* is repairable, so that in the persistence and progress of a cirrhotic state in the liver repeated infections appear to play an important role.

REFERENCES

Andrade, Z. A. (1962). Hepatic changes in advanced schistosomiasis. *Gastroenterology*, **42**, 393.

Furusawa, M. (1958). Experimental studies on the liver function in schistosomiasis japonica. *Fukuoka Acta med.*, **49**, 1158.

Hirayama, C. (1957). [Histology of the liver and changes of serum protein.] *Jap. J. Clin. exp. Med.*, **34**, 537.

Ito, T. (1971). Experimental schistosomiasis japonica: Challenge infection. *J. Kuumer med. Ass.*, **34**, 215.

Kitajima, K. (1967). Studies on the quantitative changes of serum and hepatic transaminase and alkaline phosphatase in experimental schistotomiasis japonica. *J. Kurume med. Ass.*, **30**, 64.

Matsunaga, M. (1971). Pathomorphological studies on experimental liver cirrhosis due to *Schistosoma japonicum*. *J. Kurume med. Ass.*, **34**, 1.

Miyasaka, T. (1971). Pathomorphological studies on experimental liver cirrhosis due to *Schistosoma japonicum*. *J. Kurume med. Ass.*, **34**, 34.

Nakano, H. (1969). Application of fluorescent antibody technique in experimental schistosomiasis japonica. *J. Kurume med. Ass.*, **32**, 1457.

Nakashima, T. (1971). [Liver cirrhosis due to *Schistosoma japonicum* (II): Experimental cases in animals.] *Acta hepat. jap.*, **12**, 67.

Sano, E. (1960). Quantitative changes of various serum enzymes in the experimental schistosomiasis japonica. *J. Kurume med. Ass.*, **23**, 6870.

Tsutsumi, H. (1971). Pathology of liver cirrhosis in experimental schistosomiasis japonica. *Acta path. jap.*, **21**, 156.

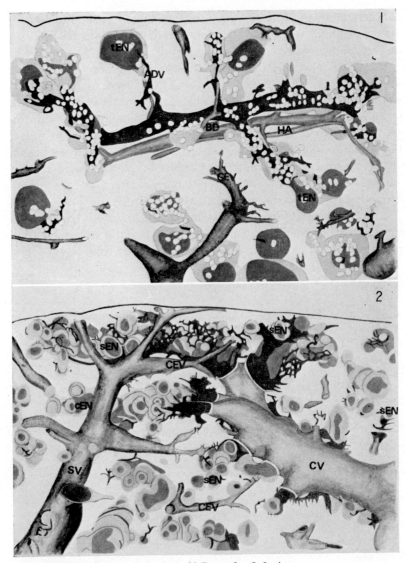

1. No. 182 (Moderate Infection), 35 Days after Infection.
    The Lesions first occur in the terminal twigs or in the axial distributing veins, and then extend to the surrounding liver paranchyma.
2. No. 60 (Moderate Infection), 38 Days after Infection.
    The egg embolism rapidly spreads towards the proximal side of the portal vein, from the terminal twig to the conducting vein. The leucocytic thrombus with matured eggs causes thrombopylephlebitis, peripylephlebitis, and portal hepatitis.

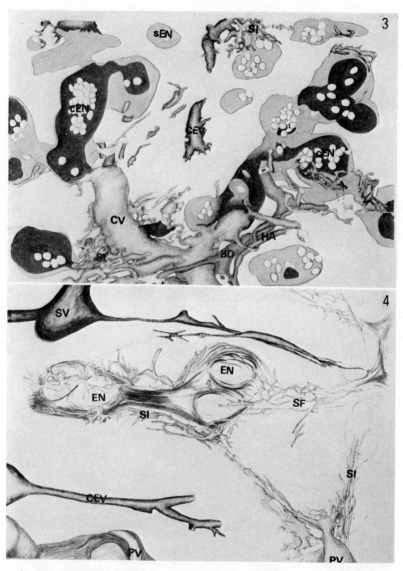

3. No. 214 (Moderate Infection), 124 Days after Infection.

Pylephlebitis and peripylephlebitis with eggs are extended to the larger conducting vein. They conglutinate with one another along a course of the portal
vein, showing a remarkable dilatation of the proximal side of the portal vein.

4. No. 13 (Slight Infection). 143 Days after Infection.

Granulomas with egg nodules in the interlobular Glisson's capsules are present.
They connect with each other with the result that the septum contains a large
number of dilated capillaries.

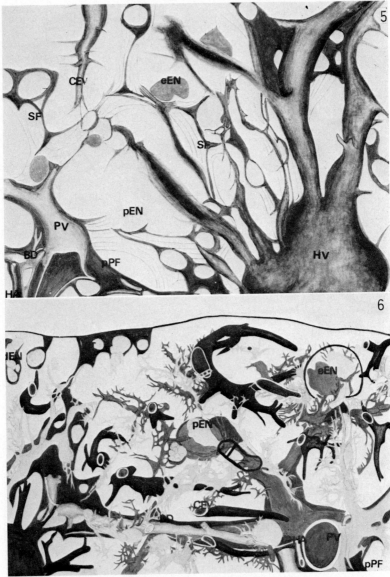

5. No. 13 (Slight Infection), 143 Days after Infection.

Besides the finding presented in Fig. 4, the wide interstitium is observed in the smaller Glisson's capsules.

6. No. 7 (Moderate Infection), 30 Weeks after Infection.

Though there are a few septums in the interlobular area, extensive connective tissues are observed below the liver capsule, together with pipe-stem fibrosis occurring in the middle-sized Glisson's capsules.

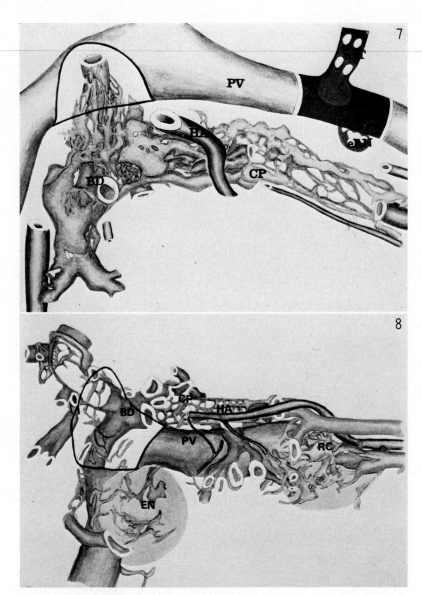

7. No. 113 (Moderate Infection Treated Incompletely).

This site corresponds to the middle-sized Glisson's capsule with a hemangiom like appearance. Dilatation of the portal vein, enlargement of the artery, and especially development of the vascular plexus in peribiliary duct are noted. Moreover, thrombopylephlebitis with eggs in the peripheral branch extends to a large portal vein present on its proximal side.

8. No. 117 (Moderate Infection Treated Incompletely, and Reinfected Later). In the interstitium with an angioma-like appearance, there are 2 large granulomas containing egg nodules: The left one is narrow in the lumen, seemingly produced extravenously on account of recovery of the vascular lumen. The right shows a progressive state of recanalization.

Figs. 9-20. Casting Patterns Showing Angiarchitecture in the Liver. Red: Artery. Yellow: Portal vein. Blue: Vena.

Fig. 9. Casting Pattern, 10 Weeks after Infection.
The entrance of resin is inhibited in the peripheral branches of the portal system.

Fig. 10. Casting Pattern, 10 Weeks after infection.
The arterial system is intensely dilated, reaching a size several times larger than normal, with a marked tortuosity.

Fig. 11. Casting Pattern, 10 Weeks after Infection.
There are collapse, deformity, and dilatation of the portal branches, on the other hand, the peripheral arterial branches are dilated, elongated, and increased in number.

Fig. 12. Casting Pattern, 20 Weeks after Infection.
The tips of the portal branches are destroyed and their proximal side is intensely dilated. Numerous branches derived from this site show a flower-like arrangement with irregular dilatation.

Figs. 13-14. Casting Patterns, 20 Weeks after Infection.
Collapse, flattening, and deformity of the portal vein, elongation and dilatation of the artery, development and dilatation of the peribiliary vascular net, and disorder of interdigitation between each vascular system are pronounced.

Figs. 15-16. Casting Patterns, 20 Weeks after Infection.
At the portion showing intense vascular changes, the smaller blood vessels with mixed color tones (arrow) consisting of the arterial and portal system are present.

Figs. 17-20. Casting Patterns, 30 Weeks after Infection.
Dilatation of the arterial system, development of the peribiliary vascular network, shortening, engorgement, and deformity of the portal vessels still remain, along with the disorder of interdigitation between each vascular system. The course of the arterial and portal system is regaining its balance.

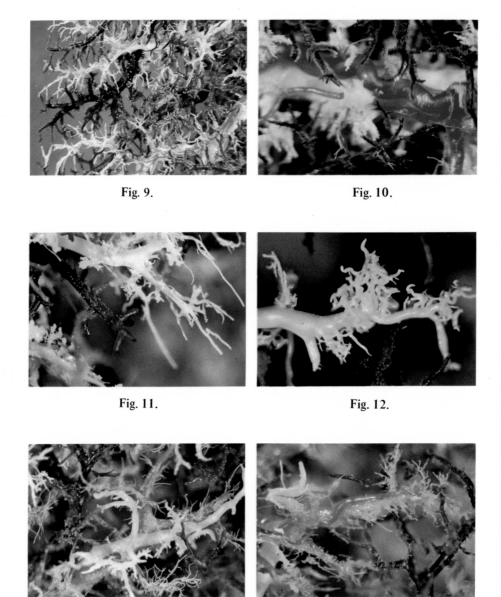

Fig. 9.

Fig. 10.

Fig. 11.

Fig. 12.

Fig. 13.

Fig. 14.

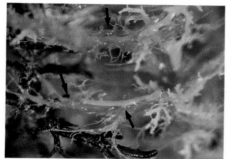

Fig. 15.

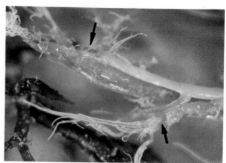

Fig. 16.

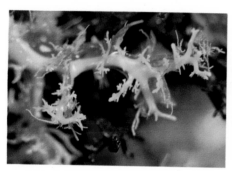

Fig. 17.

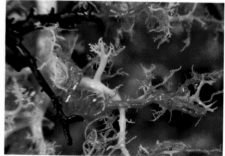

Fig. 18.

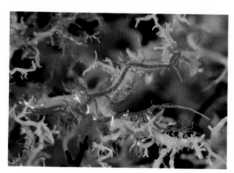

Fig. 19.

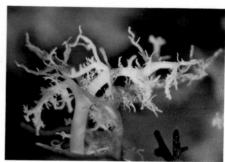

Fig. 20.

Screening of Drugs in *Schistosoma japonicum* Infections in Mice

H. Tanaka, H. Matsuda and M. Sasa

Department of Parasitology, Institute of Medical Science, University of Tokyo, Japan

INTRODUCTION

Human schistosomiasis is one of the parasitic infections that still poses problems in the world because of its wide distribution and high pathogenicity. For the treatment of this disease, such drugs as tartar emetic and related antimony compounds, lucanthone, hycanthone and niridazole have been proved effective. The extent of their practical use is, however, limited by their toxicity, and discovery of more active drugs without toxicity is anticipated, and necessary.

Screening of drugs has been done extensively in *Schistosoma mansoni* infections in mice and the techniques of the screening method have been well developed (Schubert, 1948a,b; Standen, 1953a, 1955; Pellegrino *et al.*, 1962; Pellegrino and Faria, 1965; Monteiro *et al.*, 1968; Elslager, 1971) as reviewed by Pellegrino and Katz (1969).

Use of oogram combined with change of distribution of adult schistosomes within the hepatic portal vein increased the sensitivity of screening and provided information on the mode of activity. The development of screening methods in *S. mansoni* infections in mice was due to the maintenance of *S. mansoni* in the laboratory and, consequently, of preparation of sufficient numbers of infected mice for drug testing.

A few studies have also appeared on drug testing in *S. japonicum* infections in laboratory animals (Bang and Hairston, 1946; Vogel and Minning 1948; Yokogawa *et al.*, 1969). The difficulty in experimental infections with *S. japonicum* in the laboratory remained in producing a large number of *Oncomelania* snails and in infecting them with miracidia at a high positive rate. This problem retarded the progress of drug testing with *S. japonicum*. It has remained far behind testing with *S. mansoni*.

Screening in *S. japonicum* infections is considered valuable for find-

[147]

ing drugs against *S. japonicum* since it is more resistant to drugs than is *S. mansoni*, as seen in different cure rates of drugs in the two species.

The present study was initiated to obtain a simple method for screening drugs in *S. japonicum* infections and a method for evaluating in more detail the activity of drugs which have been found in the first step of the screening.

In recent years, studies on laboratory breeding of *Oncomelania nosophora* snails (Matsuda *et al.*, 1968a,b; Matsuda, 1969; Matsuda *et al.*, 1969a,b,c; Tanaka *et al.*, 1970) and the technique of infecting snails (Matsuda *et al.*, 1970) were carried out in this laboratory. This technical progress required the production of a large number of mice infected with *S. japonicum* for studies on drug testing.

The present paper discusses the technical development of the maintenance of *S. japonicum*, basic studies on the conditions for drug testing in mice, and the results of testing chemicals and comparative efficiency of antischistosomal drugs. The methods of laboratory drug testing in *S. japonicum* infections progressed to the level of those in *S. mansoni* infections by the time the present study was prepared and new antischistosomal activity was found in a few organophorous compounds.

MATERIAL AND METHODS

Schistosoma japonicum

The schistosome used in this experiment was isolated in Kofu, Yamanashi Prefecture, Japan and maintained in dogs, mice or rabbits. This *Schistosoma* strain has been maintained in this laboratory mainly in mice and *Oncomelania nosophora* collected from Kofu and bred in this laboratory.

Infection of snails

Eggs of *Schistosoma* were obtained from the intestine of infected mice. The intestine was emulsified in physiological saline by a metal homogenizer for a few minutes and was digested with trypsin for 3 hr in a water bath at 37°C. The emulsion was strained through 2 sheets of gauze cloth, washed several times with physiological saline by centrifugation until the supernatant became clear, and washed once with 0.2% NaCl solution. This washed sediment was transferred with a pipet into the bottom of a Erlenmeyer flask which was previously filled with 0.2% NaCl solution close to the top. The flask was covered with a sheet of black paper leaving the upper narrow portion uncovered and this bare part was illuminated with an electric lamp. Miracidia floated, moving on the superficial portion of water 1 hr or more after transfer of the eggs. One hundred *Oncomelania* snails were exposed overnight to 500 miracidia in 0.2% NaCl solution in a 9 cm petri dish which was covered with wire mesh. A large watch glass was placed on the mesh to avoid the snails escaping from the water and to give sufficient exposure to miracidia (Matsuda *et al.*, 1970).

The exposed snails were kept on filter paper in a petri dish for 15 to 19 weeks. The filter paper was moistened and the snails were fed on powdered food 3 times a week. The infection rate of the snails was usually about 90% by the above method of exposure.

Infection of mice

The infected snails released an average of about 800 cercariae each by crushing. Snails were crushed with a drop of 0.2% NaCl solution between 2 glass slides and cercariae from several snails were rinsed into a small petri dish with 0.2% NaCl solution. The density of cercariae in this suspension was measured and each mouse was inoculated subcutaneously with 50 cercariae in about 0.1 ml saline using a syringe. Eggs were examined from feces of mice 6 weeks after infection and mice which were infected were provided for the drug testing.

Distribution of worms

The distribution of adult worms within the hepatic portal system was observed after the treatment. The locality of the hepatic portal system was divided into three; intrahepatic, portal and mesenteric veins. After mice were killed by extending the spinal cord, the abdominal wall and the lower part of the chest wall were opened and worms located from a part of the portal vein close to the liver to a junction of inferior mesenteric vein were collected. The worms partially entering into the liver were included in the portal vein. The liver was then taken out, pressed between two thick glass plates and the worms in it were counted under a dissecting microscope. Vessels peripheral to the portal vein were also observed and the worms found were included in the mesenteric veins. The conditions of the worms, single or paired, dead or alive, were also recorded and the distribution of worms was represented by that of females according to Standen. (1953b).

Oogram

Oogram in the intestine was observed before and after the administration of drug in mice. Oogram was first studied by Vogel (1942) in *S. japonicum* as part of embryological research and studies were developed in *S. mansoni* (Cancado, *et al.*, 1965). It has been standardized and widely applied to human diagnosis and to testing therapeutic effects of drugs in *S. mansoni* infections. In the present study, a small portion of small intestine at the middle level was removed. It was pressed on a glass slide under a cover slip by finger press and observed microscopically. The eggs in the intestinal tissue were classified into 4 stages, i.e., mature, immature, recently dead and calcified, following the standardized oogram in *S. mansoni*. Further detailed classification in immature eggs was not used.

Administration of test drugs

Test chemicals were dissolved or suspended in 10% Cremophor El and injected intraperitoneally at a dose of one fourth of half of the lethal dose daily for 4 consecutive days as a basic rule. The chemicals of which half a lethal dose was not clear were given at a dose of 100 mg/kg at first and the dose was decreased to half when mice could not tolerate the initial dose. Organophosphorous compounds were given orally.

RESULTS

1. *Distribution of worms and oogram after infection*

In order to determine an appropriate time for testing drugs in mice after infection, the distribution of females within the hepatic portal system and change of oogram in the intestine were examined continuously for a period of 4 to 14 weeks after infection. More than 110 mice were inoculated with 50 cercariae each, 10 mice were sacrificed weekly, and the distribution of females and oogram were observed. The number of females found in intrahepatic, portal and mesenteric veins was recorded in each mouse and the distribution of worms was shown by the rate, in percentage, to total females recovered.

The percent of females found in 3 parts of the hepatic portal system is illustrated in Fig. 1 by an average of 10 mice each week. The distribution of worms changed as the weeks passed. The worms as a whole tended to move from liver to mesenteric veins during this

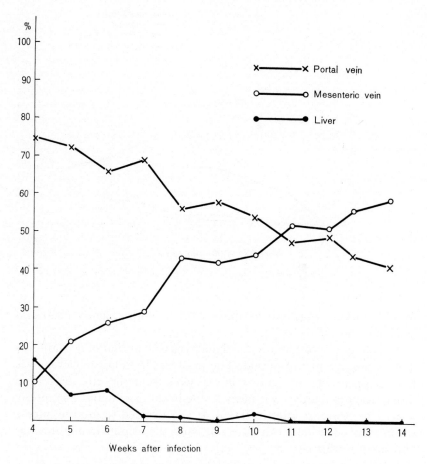

Fig. 1.   The Time Course of Distribution of Female *Schistosoma japonicum* in
Mice; Average of 10 Mice.

period. The number of females in the intrahepatic veins gradually
decreased to about 1% of total females from the 7th week after
infection. The change in the portal vein was from 75% in the 4th
week to 40% in the 14th week. In contrast, females continued to
increase in the mesenteric veins from 10% in the 4th week to 60% in
the 14th week.

   Oogram in the intestine was observed weekly in 2 mice during a
period from 5 to 12 weeks after infection. The change in rates among
4 stages of eggs is illustrated in Fig. 2. In this observation period,
rates fell from 100% to about 30% in immature eggs, rose to about

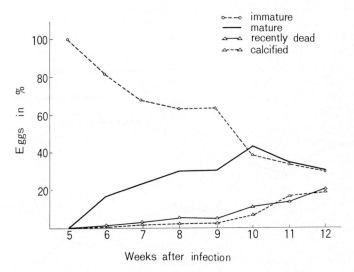

Fig. 2. Successive Change of Oogram in the Intestine after Infection. Average of 2 Mice per Week.

30% in mature eggs and to about 20% in both recently dead and calcified eggs.

The change in distribution of females as well as that of oogram was always positive in this period. The most stable trend, however, was the disappearance of females in the liver from the 7th week. The distribution of females was fairly stable in the portal and mesenteric veins 7 to 10 weeks after infection. It was decided to use the mice 7 weeks after infection for drug testing since the change in oogram was also small in this period.

2. *Change in distribution of females and oogram after treatment*

The changes in distribution of females and those of oogram after treatment have been utilized as criteria of the efficacy of drugs in *S. mansoni* infections. A hepatic shift of females usually represents change in the worm distribution within the hepatic portal system (Standen, 1953b) and the rate of mature eggs in all viable eggs stands for the change of oogram (Pellegrino, *et al.*, 1962). These changes were followed in mice infected with *S. japonicum* and treated with tartar emetic given intraperitoneally at a dose of 13 mg/kg daily for 4 consecutive days (Fig. 3).

Out of 14 mice infected, 2 mice were sacrificed daily after the treatment. The females that shifted to the liver were about 40% of total

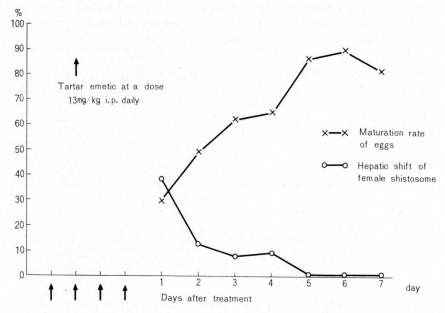

Fig. 3. Change of Hepatic Shift of Females and the Maturation Rate in Oogram of the Small Intestine after Treatment with Tartar Emetic.

females, the day after the completion of the drug administration. This hepatic shift, however, recovered abruptly on the 2nd day and disappeared 5 days after treatment. The maturation rate of eggs increased slowly until the 5th day to over 80% and remained high at 80 to 90%, as reported in *S. mansoni* infections treated with antimonial preparations (Pellegrino *et al.*, 1962).

Results of treatment with niridazole differed markedly from the above. More than 14 mice were treated with niridazole at a dose of 150 mg/kg given intraperitoneally daily for 4 days and 2 mice were sacrificed daily after the treatment (Table 1). All females that shifted to the liver on the 2nd day did not return to the portal or mesenteric veins until the 7th day. The number of mature eggs did not increase and that of immature eggs decreased slowly and disappeared from the 5th day. Coinciding with these changes, the numbers of recently dead and/or calcified eggs rose. The result appears to indicate that niridazole brings about an irreversible hepatic shift of worms, oviposition ceases and eggs not developing to maturity are killed with the mature eggs. The effect of niridazole was superior

Table 1.   The Change of Hepatic Shift of Females and Oogram in the
Small Intestine in Mice after the Termination of the Treatment with
Niridazole at a Dose of 150 mg/kg Daily for 4 Days

Days after treatment	Mouse no.	Hepatic shift (%)	Oogram in intestine (%)			
			Immat.	Mat.	R. dead	Calcif.
1	1	40	97.0	0	1.1	1.9
	2	100	85.0	1.3	9.4	4.3
2	3	100	76.7	0	22.4	0.9
	4	100	64.4	0	33.6	2.0
3	5	100	31.9	0	60.6	7.5
	6	100	2.1	0	88.5	9.4
4	7	100	13.5	0	50.5	36.0
	8	100	26.6	0	50.6	22.8
5	9	100	0	0	87.0	13.0
	10	100	0	2.4	67.2	30.4
6	11	100	0	0	64.7	35.3
	12	100	0	0	41.8	58.2
7	13	100	1.0	1.4	77.6	20.0
	14	100	0	1.1	79.7	19.2

to and quite different from that of tartar emetic which has been believed to be most effective among antimony compounds. The difference in effectiveness between the two was clearly observed from
the 5th day after the last drug administration.

The hepatic shift of females on the day after the last drug administration is an essential condition of anti-schistosomal drugs. The
technique described is applicable to the screening of a number of
test samples because of its technical simplicity. The result of hepatic
shift of females and maturation or death of eggs in the intestine shown
in the oogram on the 7th day are useful for detailed comparison of
the efficacy of drugs whose activities have been proved through the
first step of the screening.

3. Screening of drugs

To prove the technique adequate for screening, several kinds of
known anthelmintics were examined (Table 2). The infected
mice were injected intraperitoneally with a large dose of each drug
for 4 days and the distribution of females within the hepatic portal
system was observed on the day after the last drug administration.
The females shifting to the liver were nil or not significantly numerous compared with those in untreated mice when mice were treated
with thiabendazole, bithionol, diethylcarbamazine and Mel.W.

Table 2.   Distribution of Females of *S. japonicum* within the Hepatic
Portal System in Mice on the Day after Termination of the
Intraperitoneal Drug Administration for 4 Days

Drug	Daily dose mg/kg	No. of mice	Dist. of females (%)			Death rate of worms (%)
			Liver	P-vein	M-vein	
tartar emetic	13	10	10	50	40	0
	25	10	100	0	0	8
stibophen	12.5	7	41	51	8	0
	50	5	100	0	0	7
niridazole	150	6	100	0	0	33
stibnal	10	7	24	55	20	0
thiabendazole	250	10	2	42	56	0
bithionol	83.5	9	0	50	50	0
diethylcarbamazine	121.3	5	0	75	25	0
Mel W	67.5	7	2	61	37	0
Control	—	10	1	55	44	0

A significant increase in the hepatic shift was observed with tartar
emetic, stibophen, niridazole and Stibnal, especially at large doses of
the first three. The death rate of females was largest with niridazole
followed by tartar emetic and stibophen. In these comparisons, drugs
causing the hepatic shift at a rate exceeding a few percent of total
females on the day after the treatment ended could be regarded as
effective at the first step of the screening.

The infected mice were also treated by the same method with the
largest tolerable doses of 9 kinds of organophosphorous insecticides.
The distribution of females in the surviving mice among 3 mice
tested for each compound are shown in Table 3. A significant hepatic
shift was seen in dichlorvos, trichlorphon, dibrom and diazinon but
not in fentrothion, abate, malathion and fenthion. The last 4 compounds were ineffective even though mice received doses large
enough to kill 2 out of 3 mice. Diazinon was also useless because of
its high toxicity. With these considerations, the first 3 compounds
were evaluated as effective by this screening test.

The technique of the screening test was further simplified to
observe the presence of females in the liver because females rarely
shifted to the liver upon administration of ineffective drugs in the
testing. It was decided to study in detail the distribution of females
within the hepatic portal system when a few females were seen in
the liver.

A number of chemicals including various kinds out of 73 samples

Table 3. Test of Compounds Including Organophosphorus Insecticides and Niridazole in Mice Treated for 4 Consecutive Days and Sacrificed on the Day after the Last Administration

Compound	Dose mg/Kg/day	Distrib. of female %		
		Liver	P-vein	M-vein
dichlorvos	20	52.6	5.3	42.1
(DDVP)		60.0	4.0	36.0
trichlorphon	100	46.4	14.3	39.3
(dipterex)		4.3	34.8	60.9
dibrom	50	72.2	11.1	16.7
		69.0	10.3	20.7
		46.7	33.3	20.0
diazinon	5	31.8	45.5	22.7
fentrothion (Sumithion)	100	5.0	35.0	60.0
abate	100	0	100	0
malathion	100	0	100	0
fenthion (Baytex)	10	0	25.0	75.0
niridazole	100	100	0	0
		100	0	0
		100	0	0
		100	0	0
		100	0	0
73 samples		not effective		

and 7 organophosphorous compounds were tested by this simplified technique. None of the test samples were found to be effective.

4. Detailed tests of active drugs

The efficacy of the drugs for which effectiveness has been demonstrated through the first step was further studied by observing recovery of the hepatic shift of females and oogram in the intestine 7 days after the termination of treatment.

The results of the detailed test are presented in Tables 4, 5 and 6. Selected drugs were 3: tartar emetic representing the antimony compounds which are widely applied for practical human treatment, niridazole as a comparatively new drug, and dibrom which was taken from the chemicals tested in the screening discussed above. Each drug was tested at various doses diluted twofold from the largest tolerable dose.

The reaction of adult worms to the drugs was indicated by the

Table 4.   Distribution of Femal Schistosome and Oogram in the Intestine in Mice 7 Days after the Termination of Treatment with Tartar Emetic at Different Doses for 4 Consecutive Days

Tartar emetic mg/kg/ day	Mouse no.	Dist. of females %			Oogram %			
		Liver	P-vein	M-vein	Immat.	Mat.	R. dead	Calcif.
20 mg	1	60	40	0	24.8	27.7	40.0	6.8
	2	28.6	28.6	42.8	7.3	21.3	52.7	18.7
	3	11.1	66.7	22.2	10.7	43.2	38.8	7.3
	4	22.2	22.2	55.6	23.8	61.9	6.5	7.8
	5	46.1	15.4	38.5	23.8	50.0	6.2	20.0
10 mg	1	0	30.8	69.2	6.3	45.4	28.3	20.0
	2	0	33.3	66.7	11.7	54.5	23.4	10.4
	3	0	13.3	86.7	4.0	77.0	15.0	4.0
	4	11.1	33.3	55.6	19.7	77.0	0.3	3.0
	5	0	25.0	75.0	17.6	75.9	1.0	5.5
5 mg	1	0	33.3	66.7	30.3	22.0	41.4	6.3
	2	0	50.0	50.0	28.7	50.7	20.3	0.3
	3	0	18.8	72.2	22.1	42.5	26.5	8.9
	4	0	44.4	55.6	49.6	38.7	4.7	7.0
	5	0	20.0	80.0	34.3	38.7	11.3	15.7
2.5 mg	1	0	18.2	81.8	58.7	27.3	13.3	0.7
	2	0	41.7	58.3	30.6	56.8	11.3	1.3
	3	0	37.5	62.5	72.3	20.7	4.3	2.7
	4	0	25.0	75.0	47.1	33.8	7.7	11.4
	5	0	57.1	42.9	69.0	16.0	8.0	7.0

distribution of females and the action of drugs to oviposition and to eggs was analyzed by comparing oograms in tested mice with those of untreated mice (Tables 5 and 6).

In the test with tartar emetic (Table 4), the hepatic shift was recovered or did not occur at doses of 10 mg/kg or less, and was not recovered in 20 mg group. The oviposition was notably limited in 20 and 10 mg groups. The maturation rates of eggs increased also in these 2 groups especially at a dose of 10 mg/kg. More eggs were killed in large dose groups.

The action of niridazole presented more striking reactions to adults and eggs (Table 5). The hepatic shift remained, oviposition ceased and eggs were killed without maturation at a dose of 150 mg/kg. This kind of reaction has not been observed at 20 mg/kg or at the tolerable largest dose of tartar emetic. The rate of hepatic shift remained high in the 100 mg group, the oviposition was more

Table 5.   Distribution of Female Schistosome and Oogram in the Intestine in Mice 7 Days after the Termination of Treatment with Niridazole at Different Doses for 4 Consecutive Days

Niridazole mg/kg		Dist. of females %			Oogram in intestine (%)			
		Liver	P-vein	M-vein	Immat.	Mat.	R. dead	Calcif.
150	1	100	0	0	4.2	1.6	15.1	79.0
	2	100	0	0	12.6	1.1	1.3	85.0
	3	100	0	0	4.4	0	0.9	94.7
100	1	100	0	0	6.0	28.3	30.7	35.0
	2	50	25	25	18.1	34.8	25.4	21.7
	3	77.8	11.1	11.1	16.3	26.0	37.7	20.0
	4	87.5	12.5	0	2.7	27.0	37.3	33.0
50	1	0	12.5	87.5	13.0	29.0	32.0	26.0
	2	0	20.7	79.3	24.3	52.4	16.0	7.3
	3	0	33.3	66.7	22.7	47.0	19.0	11.3
	4	0	18.5	81.5	7.7	71.6	9.0	11.7
	5	0	40.0	60.0	12.3	60.0	12.7	15.0
25	1	0	25.7	74.3	21.3	60.0	7.7	11.0
	2	0	44.4	55.6	35.3	53.0	8.0	3.7
	3	0	22.2	77.8	35.3	56.4	3.3	5.0
	4	0	71.4	28.6	70.1	22.1	4.6	3.2
	5	0	40.0	60.0	61.7	28.3	9.6	0.4
Control	1	0	40.0	60.0	67.8	23.3	4.8	4.1
	2	0	60.0	40.0	68.4	26.5	1.3	3.8
	3	0	33.3	66.7	67.7	22.6	4.3	5.4
	4	0	60.0	40.0	64.2	31.1	1.8	2.9
	5	0	66.7	33.3	69.1	21.5	1.7	7.7

limited and death rates of eggs rose in proportion to the increase of doses. The hepatic shift at a 100 mg dose of niridazole and the oogram at a 50 mg dose corresponded approximately to those at 20 mg of tartar emetic.

The efficacy of dibrom was not as conspicuous as that of the 2 drugs shown in Table 6. The hepatic shift was largely recovered at the largest dose or 50 mg/kg. The limitation of oviposition, increase of maturation rate and rise of death rate of eggs were observed at doses of 50 and 25 mg/kg. The degree of these changes, however, was not as large when compared with values in the control group, and there was a large individual variation among mice in each dose group. The action of dibrom at 50 mg/kg in adults was inferior to that of tartar emetic at 20 mg/kg. The action of dibrom in oogram was similar to that of tartar emetic at 10 mg/kg.

Table 6. Distribution of Female Schistosome and Oogram in the Intestine in Mice 7 Days after the Termination of Treatment with Dibrom at Different Doses for 4 Consecutive Days

Dibrom mg/Kg/ day	Mouse no.	Dist. of females %			Oogram (%)			
		Liver	P-vein	M-vein	Immat.	Mat.	R. dead	Calcif.
50 mg	1	0	0	100	13.3	80.4	6.3	0
	2	0	50	50	26.3	56.7	10.0	7.0
	3	14.3	14.3	71.4	32.3	33.0	31.0	3.7
	4	25.0	25.0	50.0	24.0	46.0	20.0	10.0
	5	0	0	100	75.3	8.0	7.0	9.7
25 mg	1	0	22.2	77.8	29.0	58.0	4.7	8.3
	2	0	87.5	12.5	23.3	17.7	36.7	22.3
	3	0	16.7	83.3	55.0	34.0	8.0	3.0
	4	0	64.7	35.3				
	5	0	33.3	66.7	69.0	21.0	6.7	3.3
12.5 mg	1	0	66.7	33.3	38.0	27.7	20.0	14.3
	2	0	100	0	38.7	50.6	10.0	0.7
	3	0	50	50	64.0	16.0	15.3	4.7
	4	6.7	53.3	40.0	56.0	38.7	2.3	3.0
	5	0	28.6	71.4	64.4	27.3	4.0	4.3
Control	1	0	40.0	60.0	67.8	23.3	4.8	4.1
	2	0	60.0	40.0	68.4	26.5	1.3	3.8
	3	0	33.3	66.7	67.7	22.6	4.3	5.4
	4	0	60.0	40.0	64.2	31.1	1.8	2.9
	5	0	66.7	33.3	69.1	21.5	1.7	7.7

The degree of efficacy of each drug was thus demonstrated by observing the distribution of females and oograms in the intestine.

DISCUSSION

Success in establishing methods for testing drugs in mice infected with *S. japonicum* in the present study was based on the laboratory breeding of *Oncomelania nosophora* and infecting them with miracidia at high positive rates. The method of breeding was as follows: Adult snails were reared on a wet soil surface in pottery and fed on powdered food (Matsuda, 1969). Under these conditions, the average progeny produced per female per month was 54.6 in the Kofu strain of *Oncomelania* snails (Tanaka *et al.*, 1971). The young snails were transferred into a water tank in which soil was placed at the bottom, water was aerated and cut pieces of rice straw and filter paper were provided as nutrient. Young snails, 0.5 mm in length, developed into adults of 5 mm in 2 months (Matsuda, 1969).

The method for obtaining comparatively pure eggs of *Schistosoma* from mouse intestine was useful in providing active miracidia which produced high infection rates among *Oncomelania* snails. The method infecting snails in 0.2% NaCl solution (Matsuda *et al.* 1970) was also useful.

S. mansoni in mice has been widely used for chemotherapeutic studies on schistosomiasis. The patterns of fecal discharge of eggs, survival time of treated mice, distribution of adult worms within the hepatic portal system and oogram changes were extensively studied. These changes have been used as criteria in the evaluation of anti-schistosomal drugs. Among these criteria, distribution of worms and oogram were taken into consideration in the present study of *S. japonicum* for the simplicity of techniques involved and for satisfactory results.

In the distribution of adult *S. japonicum* within the hepatic system in mice, the worms in the intrahepatic veins reached a minimum level after the 7th week as reported in *S. mansoni* infections in mice by Standen (1953a). The drug testing was initiated 7 weeks after infection since the death rate of the infected mice increased from the 8th week. The shift of worms to the liver was represented by the females according to Standen (1953b). The test drugs were regarded as effective when no worms were found in the liver after the treatment. In that case, examination for detailed distribution was not carried out. The hepatic shift of females 5 days after the initiation of drug administration was valuable in evaluating the drug activity.

The reduction in the first stage of immature eggs was reported to be a reliable criterion for drug screening (Pellegrino *et al.*, 1962), but this technique was more complicated than observation of the hepatic shift as a routine procedure at the primary step of the screening.

The embryological development of eggs was first studied in *S. japonicum* by Vogel (1942) and the change of development of eggs by the treatment was reported by Bang and Hairston (1946). These findings were developed into the oogram system, and oogram change was applied to drug testing in *S. mansoni* by Pellegrino *et al.* (1962), Pelligrino and Faria (1965) and Cancado *et al.*, (1965).

In oogram change, decrease in the first stage of immature eggs and increase in maturation rates were reported useful for criteria of drug activity. The increase of the death rate of eggs has so far been regarded as the result of decrease in immature eggs or cessation of oviposition. This rate, however, added its own significance after niridazole was found to actively kill eggs (Monteiro *et al.*, 1968).

Accordingly, eggs in the intestine were placed into 4 stages in the present study: immature, mature, recently dead and calcified. This was to indicate cessation of oviposition, increase in maturation and in death rate.

The hepatic shift of worms and the change of oogram remained until 7 days after termination of drug administration when the test drugs were as active as those widely used for human treatment. These observations were applied to detailed testing of drugs in varying doses. The change of oogram was not only a sensitive criterion of drug activity but also provided information about the mode of action and degree of activity of test drugs. New chemical compounds were tested as well as those already known by this screening schedule and the degree of activity in known active drugs were well presented. The activity was also demonstrated in a group of organophosphorous compounds especially in dichlorovos, trichlorphon and dibrom. The activity of the first 2 compounds was reported by Cerf *et al.* (1962), Talaat *et al.* (1966) and Hass (1969). Activity of dibrom was newly found in the present study. Promising results will be expected in the future in the testing of organophosphorous compounds.

SUMMARY

An attempt was made to standardize the method of drug screening in *Schistosoma japonicum* infections in mice. For this purpose, a large number of *Oncomelania nosophora* infected with *Schistosoma japonicum* were produced in the laboratory using *Oncomelania* snails cultured in the laboratory. High infection rates of 90% or more in snails were obtained. The change of distribution of *Schistosoma* within the hepatic portal system in mice and that of oogram in intestine followed the infection. On this observation, drug administration was initiated in the 7th week after infection since worms usually moved out of the liver and the pattern of oogram was comparatively stable at this time. The drugs were mainly given intraperitoneally at 1/4 of LD 50 to the largest tolerable dose daily for 4 consecutive days. For the first step of screening, the hepatic shift of females on the day after the termination of treatment was found to be a sensitive and satisfactory criterion for evaluating test drugs having the advantage of simple procedures in the technique. Out of 8 known anthelmintics, antischistosomal activity was proven in tartar emetic, stibophen, stibnal and niridazole. Activity was also observed in dichlorvos, trichlorphon, dibrom and diazinon out of 8 samples of organophosphorous insecticides. No efficacy was observed in the other 73 chemical samples. The degree of antischistosomal activity and the mode of action of active drugs were demonstrated in detail by observing the recovery of the hepatic shift and the change of oogram in the intestine 1 week after the termination of drug administration. Comparing 3 representative active drugs, niridazole showed the strongest activity, followed by stibophene and dibrom. Niridazole was found to actively kill the worms and eggs, and the efficacy of dibrom was inferior to stibophen.

REFERENCES

Bang, F. B. and Hairston, N. G. (1946). Studies on schistosomiasis IV. Chemotherapy of experimental schistosomiasis japonica. *Am. J. Hyg.*, **44**, 348.

Cancado, J. R., Cunha, A. S., Carvalho, D. G. and Cambraia (1965). Evaluation of the treatment of human *Schistosoma mansoni* infection by the quantitative oogram technique. *Bull. WHO*, **33**, 557.

Cerf, J., Lebrun, A. and Dierichx, J. (1962). A new approach to helminthiasis control: The use of an organophosphorous compound. *Am. J. Trop. Med. Hyg.*, **11**, 514.

Elslager, E. F. (1971). Chemotherapy of schistosomiasis: Progress at a snail's pace. *Japanese J. Trop. Med.*, **11**, 34.

Hass, D. K. (1969). Oaganophophorous compounds and parasite chemotherapy. Working paper presented to the meeting of the US-Japan Cooperative Medical Science Program.

Matsuda, H. (1969). Studies on experimental schistosomiasis. 1. Studies on the methods for mass breeding of the snail intermediate host, *Oncomelania hupensis nosophora*. *Japan. J. Parasit.*, **18**, 523. (Japanese article with English summary)

Matsuda, H., Kobayashi, J. and Sasa, M. (1968a). Studies on the laboratory mass-breeding of *Oncomelania* snails. *Japan. J. Parasit.*, **17**, 283. (Ab. in Japanese)

Matsuda, H., Sasa, M. and Kobayashi, J. (1968b). Further studies on the laboratory breeding of *Oncomelania snails*, the intermediate hosts of *Schistosoma japonicum*. *Japan. J. Parasit.*, **17**, 570. (Ab. in Japanese)

Matsuda, H., Kobayashi, J. and Sasa, M. (1969). Further studies on the laboratory breeding of *Oncomelania* snails, the intermediate host of *Schistosoma japonicum*. *Japan. J. Trop. Med.*, **10**, 95 (Ab.).

Matsuda, H., Kudo, Y. and Hashiguchi, J. (1969a). Laboratory observations on the egg production of *Oncomelania* snails under various conditions. *Japan. J. Parasit.*, **18**, 662. (Ab. in Japanese)

Matsuda H., Hashiguchi, J., Kudo, Y. and Sasa, M. (1969b). Mass culture of *Oncomelania* snails in the laboratory. *Japan. J. Parasit.*, **18**, 662. (Ab. in Japanese)

Matsuda, H., Hashiguchi, J. and Sasa, M. (1970). Susceptibility and cercarial formation in *Oncomelania* snails to *Schistosoma japonicum. Japan. J. Parasit.*, **19**, 359 (Ab. in Japanese)

Monteiro, W., Pellegrino, J. and Henriques da Silva, M. L. (1968). Unusual oogram pattern in mice after niridazole treatment. *J. Parasit.*, **54**, 175.

Pellegrino, J. and Faria, J. (1965). The oogram method for the screening of drugs in schistosomiasis mansoni. *Am. J. Trop. Med. Hyg.*, **14**, 363–369.

Pellegrino, J. and Katz, N. (1969). Laboratory evaluation of antischistosomal agents. *Ann. N.Y. Acad. Sci.*, **160**, 429.

Pellegrino, J., Oliveira, C. A., Faria, J. and Cunha, A. S. (1962). New approach to the screening of drugs in experimental schistosomiasis mansoni in mice. *Am. J. Trop. Med. Hyg.*, **11**, 20.

Schubert, M. (1948a). Conditions for drug testing in experimental schistosomiasis mansoni in mice. *Am. J. Trop. Med.*, **28**, 121.

Schubert, M. (1948b). Screening of drugs in experimental schistosomiasis mansoni in mice. *Am. J. Trop. Med.*, **28**, 137.

Standen, O. D. (1953a). Experimental schistosomiasis. III. Chemotherapy and mode of drug action. *Ann. Trop. Med. Parasit.*, **47**, 26.

Standen, O. D. (1953b). The relationship of sex in *Schistosoma mansoni* to migration within the hepatic portal system of experimentally infected mice. *Ann. Trop. Med. Parasit.*, **47**, 139.

Standen, O. D. (1955). The treatment of experimental schistosomiasis in mice: sexual maturity and drug response. *Ann. Trop. Med. Parasit.*, **49**, 183.

Talaat, S. M., Amin, N. and El-Masry, B. (1966). A comparative study of Dipterex and tartar emetic in the treatment of urinary schistosomiasis. *Trans. Roy Soc. Trop. Med. Hyg.*, **60**, 579.

Tanaka, H., Matsuda, H., Nihei, N. and Sasa, M. (1971). Basic studies for screening tests of drugs against *Schistosoma japonicum. Japan. J. Trop. Med.*, **11**, 37.

Yokogawa, M., Sano, M. and Kojima, S. (1969). Chemotherapy with hycanthone for the experimentally infected animals with *Schistosoma japonicum. Japan. J. Parasit.*, **18**, 416 (Ab. in Japanese)

Vogel, H. (1942). Über Entwicklung, Lebensdauer und Tod der Eier von *Bilharzia japonica* im Wirtsgewe. *Deutsche Tropenmedizinische Zeitschrift.*, **46**, 57–69, 81.

Vogel, H. and Minning, W. (1948). The action of Miracil in *Schistosoma japonicum* infection in laboratory animals. *Ann. Trop. Med. Parasit.*, **42**, 268.

Studies on the Immuno-Diffusion Tests of
Schistosoma japonicum

M. Tsuji* and M. Yokogawa**

*Department of Parasitology, School of Medicine,
Hiroshima University, Hiroshima, Japan
**Department of Parasitology, School of Medicine,
Chiba University, Chiba, Japan

INTRODUCTION

The control of schistosomiasis japonica is an important problem among the parasitic diseases in Japan. It involves, basically, survey and mass treatment for schistosomiasis. Until recently, most of the surveys for schistosomiasis in an endemic area were made by stool examination, but the recovery of eggs in stools is sometimes difficult in light cases or therapeutically affected cases.

A considerable amount of work on the methods of immunological diagnosis has been reported in recent years (Biguet *et al.*, 1967; Capron *et al.*, 1966; Yokogawa *et al.*, 1968; Tsuji, 1971). However, the practical value of such tests as the intradermal test, complement fixation test, agglutination test and circum oval precipitin test for a screening method for schistosomiasis or criterion of cure after treatment has not yet been ascertained.

Recently, the Ouchterlony test and immunoelectrophoresis have produced promising results for the differentiation of certain species of helminths, as well as for immunological diagnosis of helminthic diseases (Biguet *et al.*, 1962; Kagan and Norman, 1963; Kent, 1963; Tsuji, 1968; Tsuji *et al.*, 1967, 1968).

The authors applied immuno-diffusion tests to the diagnosis of schistosomiasis, and some interesting results were obtained.

METHOD

Immuno-diffusion tests for *Schistosoma japonicum* on agar plate were performed by the Ouchterlony method and immunoelectrophoresis (Grabar and Burtin, 1964; Tsuji, 1968). As antigen, 0.1% saline extract of the adult worms of *S. japonicum* was used, and 0.9% Marque Agarose in veronal buffered saline (pH 8.2) was used. This buffer solution is prepared from 160 grams of sodium veronal dissolved in distilled water (to make 10 liters), adding 220 ml of 1 N hydrochloric acid to bring the pH to 8.2.

RESULTS

1) *Studies of immunoelectrophoresis on the cross reactions between* S. japonicum *and other trematodes with immunized rabbit sera*

In this study, rabbit anti-serum immunized with *S. japonicum* and antigens of 7 species of trematodes, and reverse combination of antigen and antiserum were used for immunoelectrophoresis.

The results are as shown in Table 1. The serum of rabbit immunized with *S. japonicum* showed 23 bands with *S. japonicum* antigen, and its immunoelectrophoresis diagram is as shown in Fig. 1.

The number of bands demonstrable in the case of immunization with *S. japonicum* with various antigens were 11 bands with *S. mansoni* antigen, 4 bands each with *Fasciola hepatica*, *Clonorchis sinensis*, *Paragonimus westermani* and *P. miyazakii* antigens, and 3 bands with *P. ohirai* antigen.

The reverse, *i.e.*, the relations between *S. japonicum* antigen and the rabbit sera immunized with other trematodes were almost parallel to those shown in Table 1. Namely, the *S. japonicum* antigen showed 11 bands with the imunized rabbit serum with *S. mansoni*, 4 bands each with the anti-sera with *F. hepatica* and *C. sinensis*, 2 bands each with *P. westermani* and *P. ohirai* and 1 band with *P. miyazakii* anti-sera.

The results of our experiences with Capron in the cross reactions among various helminths by immunoelectrophoresis are summarized in Table 2. It can be said from the results that some common bands of trematodes do exist, and the strongest reactions were observed between the antigen and its homologous anti-sera.

2) *Studies of the Ouchterlony test for schistosomiasis japonica patients*

The Ouchterlony test was performed on the sera of 83 patients with *S. japonicum*. Eighty-one cases (97.6%) out of 83 showed the existence of precipitating antibodies, and from 1 to 6 bands were noticed.

Cross reactions in the Ouchterlony test was perfomed on the 10 cases among these whose sera had antigens of 4 other kinds of helminths and C-reactive protein. The results are shown in Table 3.

Table 1. Cross Reactions between *Schistosoma japonicum* and Other Helminths with Immunized Rabbit Sera by Immunoelectrophoresis

	S. japonicum	S. mansoni	F. hepatica	C. sinensis	P. westermani	P. ohirai	P. miyazakii
Antigens							
Immunized rabbit sera with S. japonicum	23	11	4	4	4	3	4
Immunized rabbit sera							
Antigen of S. japonicum	23	11	4	4	2	2	1

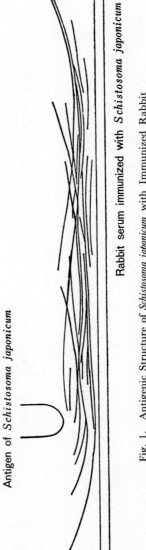

Antigen of *Schistosoma japonicum*

Rabbit serum immunized with *Schistosoma japonicum*

Fig. 1. Antigenic Structure of *Schistosoma japonicum* with Immunized Rabbit
Serum by Means of Immunoelectrophoresis.

Table 2. Cross Reactions among Various Parasitic Helminths

0.1 % NaCl extract antigens	Immunized Rabbit Sera													
	F.h.	D.d.	C.s.	P.w.	P.m.	P.o.	S.m.	S.h.	S.j.	T.s.	H.n.	A.s.	T.c.	Anis.
Trematoda														
Fasciola hepatica	25	6	5	5	4	5	5	5	4	5	2	2	0	0
Dicrocoelium dendriticum	6	19	5	5	5	5	3	3	2				0	0
Clonorchis sinensis	5	5	21	5	5	5	5	5	4			0	0	0
Opisthorchis felineus	4	3	11	4			2	2	1			0		
Paragonimus westermani	6	5	5	23	14	14	4	4	4	2	1	0	0	0
Paragonimus miyazakii	4	4	5	13	22	13	3		4	2	1	0	0	0
Paragonimus ohirai	4	4	4	13	13	22	3	3	3	1	1	0	0	0
Schistosoma mansoni	5	3	5	4	3	3	21	19	11	5	1	2	0	0
Schistosoma haematobium	5	3	5	4			19	21	11	1				
Schistosoma japonicum	4	2	4	2	2	2	11	11	23	2	1	2	0	
Cestoidea														
Tenia saginata	5			1	1	1	5		2	24	6	2	0	0
Hymenolepsis nana	2			1	1	1	1		1	6	21	2	0	0
Nematoda														
Ascaris suum	2	0	0	0	0	0	2		2	2	2	24	13	12
Toxocara canis	0	0	0	0	0	0	1		1	0	0	13	23	12
Anisakis larvae	0	0	0	0	0	0	0		0	0	0	12	12	24

Table 3.   Cross Reactions in Immuno-diffusion Tests for Schistosomiasis japonica (Tsuji, 1971)

0.1 % NaCl extract Antigens	Case No.										No. posit. No.exam.(%)
	1	2	3	4	5	6	7	8	9	10	
Ouchterlony											
S. japonicum	2	2	5	2	4	5	4	2	3	3	10/10 (100)
S. mansoni	0	2	3	0	2	2	2	0	2	1	7/10 (70)
F. hepatica	0	1	0	0	0	1	0	0	0	0	2/10 (20)
P. westermani	0	1	0	0	0	1	0	0	0	1	3/10 (30)
A. lumbricoides	0	0	0	0	0	0	0	0	0	0	0/10 (0)
C R P	1	0	1	1	1	1	1	1	1	1	9/10 (90)
I. E. P.											
S. japonicum	3	3	5	2	6	5	5	2	3	5	10/10 (100)
S. mansoni	1	2	3	0	2	2	3	0	2	1	8/10 (80)

Seven cases out of 10 showed 1 to 3 bands with *S. mansoni* antigen, 2 cases with *F. hepatica* antigen and 3 cases with the antigen of *P. westermani* showed 1 band, but the antigen of *Ascaris lumbricoides* did not show any reaction with those sera of schistosomiasis japonica patients.

The studies on the practical value of the Ouchterlony test for schistosomiasis as a criterion of cure were carried out on 44 schistosomiasis japonica patients for two years after treatment with Niridazol. The results showed that 24 cases out of 44 remained negative for *S. japonicum* eggs for two years after treatment. However, only 6 out of 24 egg-negative cases were found to be negative with the Ouchterlony test. Further observations with stool examination and immuno-diffusion tests are being carried out on other cases who received treatment with Niridazol in Yamanashi prefecture.

Determining whether or not cure for schistosomiasis has been effective is very difficult in patients inhabiting the endemic area. Reinfection with *S. japonicum* cannot be excluded among these individuals. However, the numbers of precipitin bands in the Ouchterlony test of the patients who had been treated with Niridazol showed a tendency to decrease after treatment in the cases mentioned above.

The Ouchterlony reaction is closely correlated with the patient, and should be a very useful method of immuno-diagnosis for schistosomiasis, from the above-mentioned results (97.6%). Further, it might be possible to evaluate the efficacy of the treatment on the basis of comparative studies on the results of Ouchterlony tests before, during and after treatment.

3) *Studies of immunoelectrophoresis on schistosomiasis japonica*

After preliminary studies by means of the Ouchterlony method, the sera of 21 patients infected with *S. japonicum* in an endemic area of Yamanashi Prefecture were tested by immunoelectrophoresis. In immunoelectrophoresis all patients showed 2 to 11 bands with *S. japonicum* antigen.

The sera of 10 cases of these were also tested with the antigen of *S. mansoni*. Seven cases out of 10 showed a weak reaction with *S. mansoni* antigen, and the number of bands were from 1 to 3 as illustrated in Table 3.

The immunoelectrophoretic diagrams are shown in Figs. 2 and 3. It can be said from these diagrams that band No. 1 is the common precipitation of the genus *Schistosoma*, and band No. 2 is the specific precipitation for schistosomiasis japonica.

Band No. 1 which is markedly curved and formed close to the antibody trough demonstrated both antigens of *S. japonicum* and *S. mansoni*. Band No. 2 which is slightly curved and situated far from the trough reflected strong reactivity in all cases of schistosomiasis japonica patients. The interpretation of such patterns is very difficult and may be resolved by repeating the experiment with the absorption technique. The absorption technique should be handled with care. One ml of the hyper-immune rabbit serum of *S. japonicum* was absorbed with 20 mg of another antigen (for example, *S. mansoni* antigen). After stirring, the antiserum-antigen mixture was incubated for 3 hr at 37°C and then stored in the refrigerator for 12–24 hours. Band No. 2 was recognized as the residual reaction of anti-*S. japonicum* serum after absorption. Figure 4 shows the immunoelectrophoretic diagram of schistosomiasis japonica patient serum by the trough cut method. A comparison of the relative positions of the bands which develop may identify the antigen. Band No. 1 of both antigens of *S. japonicum* and *S. mansoni* were joined at the positive side of electrode, and this band is the common precipitation of schistosome.

4) *Studies of antigenic communities between host and parasite*

The studies on antigenic communities were carried out by the use of rabbit serum immunized with *S. japonicum* and extracts of snails by immunoelectrophoresis. The results are as shown in Table 4.

In the case of immunization with *S. japonicum*, 4 bands were seen with *Oncomelania nosophora* antigen as shown in Fig. 5, 1 band each with *Bulinus truncatus* and *Biomphalaria pfeifferi* antigens, and none

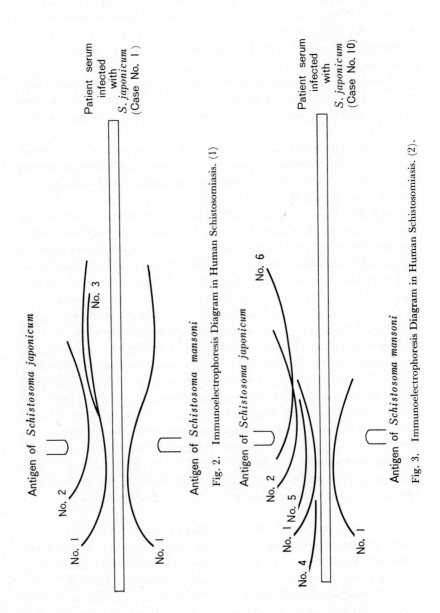

Fig. 2. Immunoelectrophoresis Diagram in Human Schistosomiasis. (1)

Fig. 3. Immunoelectrophoresis Diagram in Human Schistosomiasis. (2).

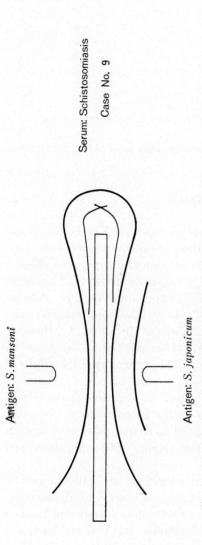

Antigen: *S.mansoni*

Serum: Schistosomiasis

Case No. 9

Antigen: *S. japonicum*

Fig. 4. Immunoelectrophoresis Diagram in Human Schistosomiasis by the Trough Cut Method.

Antigen *Oncomelania nosophora*

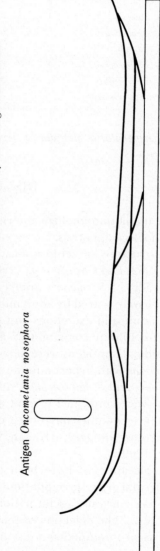

Rabbit serum immunized with *Schistosoma japonicum*

Fig. 5. Immunoelectrophoresis Diagram between *Schistosoma japonicum* and *Oncomelania nosophora*.

Table 4.   Cross Reactions between Parasites and Intermediate-hosts

Antigens	Immunized rabbit sera					
	S.j.	S.m.	P.w.	P.m.	P.o.	F.h.
Biomphalaria glabrata	0	4	1	0	0	0
Bulinus truncatus	1	0	0	0	0	0
Lymnaea truncatula	0	0	0	0	0	5
Melania libertina	0	0	4	0	0	1
Oncomelania nosophora	4	0	0	0	1	0
Biomphalaria pfeifferi	1	3	1	0	0	0
Pila scutata gracilis			0	0	0	0

with *Biomphalaria glabrata*, *Lymnaea truncatula* and *Melania libertina* antigens.

DISCUSSION

The use of immunological techniques, especially Ouchterlony and immunoelectrophoresis, has revealed the great complexity of the antigenic structure of schistosome. By immunoelectrophoresis, Biguet *et al.* (1962) and Capron *et al.* (1965, 1966) demonstrated 21 antigens in extracts of *S. mansoni* adults using hyper-immune sera. Among them 11 were shared by adult and egg, 14 by adult and cercariae, and 12 by adult and excretions and secretions of the worm. Of these 21 antigens, 19 were common to *S. haematobium* and 10 to *S. japonicum*. In our study, 23 antigens were demonstrated in extracts of the adults of *S. japonicum* with hyper-immune serum, and 11 each were common to *S. mansoni* and *S. haematobium*, and some common precipitins (1 to 4 bands) were confirmed present among the trematodes.

Many techniques have been derived to detect antibodies against schistosome antigens. (Kagan, 1958; Kent, 1963; Smithers and Terry, 1969)

Soluble antigens have been used to detect antibodies active in intradermal tests, precipitation reactions of several kinds, complement fixation tests, agglutination and flocculation tests and fluorescence tests. The detection of these antibodies was carried out in the interests of immunodiagnosis. Antibodies of schistosome also react with every stages of parasites; cercarienhüllen reaction, cercarial agglutination, miracidial immobilization, circumoval precipitin test and fluorescent antibody reactions.

The authors applied to the diagnosis for schistosomiasis japonica the immuno-diffusion tests (Ouchterlony and Immunoelectrophoresis). These tests do not cover a sufficient number of cases, but it seems that the Ouchterlony test is closely correlated with patients' sera (97.6%) and the immunoelectrophoresis has a perfect response to the antigen of *S. japonicum* (100%). Further, both techniques are useful method for the diagnosis of schistosomiasis japonica.

The antibody response to the treatment with Niridazol is now being studied in individuals in an endemic area of schistosomiasis in Yamanashi Prefecture and promising results are expected. It might be possible to evaluate the efficacy of the treatment from comparative studies on the results before, during and after treatment in the Ouchterlony test and immunoelectrophoresis.

In this study, the Ouchterlony test and immunoelectrophoresis were successfully performed on cases of schistosomiasis japonica patients and this may indicate that the tests would be useful methods for the diagnosis of schistosomiasis japonica. It can also be said that immunological diagnosis for schistosomiasis should be conducted simultaneously with the Ouchterlony test, immunoelectrophoresis and other immunological techniques.

On the study of antigenic communities between host and parasite, the presence of antigens in extracts of homogenized schistosomes indistinguishable from antigens of the vertebrate host, has been reported by Damian (1967). Using immuno-diffusion techniques, Damian demonstrated at least 4 common antigens between schistosome homogenate and the albino mouse serum in which the schistosomes were grown. Capron *et al.* (1965, 1968), using the immunoelectrophoretic method, identified 5 antigenic fractions common to *S. mansoni* and the liver from the hamster in which these worms were grown, and 2 of these antigens could be identified in man. They were also able to demonstrate the persistence in the adult worm of antigens which were common to the intermediate host, *B. glabrata*. In our study, 4 bands were demonstrated between immunized rabbit serum with *S. japonicum* and *O. nosophora*.

CONCLUSION

The Ouchterlony test and immunoelectrophoresis were applied to diagnosis for schistosomiasis japonica.

1) Twenty-three antigens were demonstrated in extract of *S. japo-*

nicum adults with hyper-immune serum, and 11 each were common to genus *schistosoma*, and some common precipitins (1 to 4 bands) were demonstrated among the trematodes.

2) Eighty-one cases (97.6%) out of 83 schistosomiasis japonica cases showed the existence of precipitating antibodies by the Ouchterlony test, and the number of bands noticed were between 1 and 6.

3) In immunoelectrophoresis, all of 21 schistosomiasis japonica patients showed 2 to 11 bands with *S. japonicum* antigen.

4) On the antigenic communities between host and parasite, 4 bands were demonstrable between immunized rabbit serum with *S. japonicum* and intermediate host, *O. nosophora*.

REFERENCES

Biguet, J., Capron, A. and Tran Van Ky, P. (1962).   Les antigènes de *Schistosoma mansoni*. I. Étude électrophorétique et immunoélectrophrétique. Caractérisation des antigènes spécifiques. *Ann. Inst. Past.*, **103**, 763.

Biguet, J., Capron, A. and Tran Van Ky, P. (1967).   Le diagnostic immunologique des parasitoses humaines. *Lille Médical.*, **12**, 43.

Capron, A., Biguet, J., Rosé, F. and Vernes, A. (1965).   Les antigènes de *Schistosoma mansoni*. II. Étude immunoélectrophorétique comparée de divers stade larvaires et des adultes de deux sexes. Aspects immunologiques des relations hôte-parasite de la cercaire et de l'adulte de *S. mansoni*. *Ann. Inst. Past.*, **109**, 798.

Capron, A., Vernes, A., Biguet, J. and Rosé, F. (1966).   Les précipitines sériques dans les Bilharziosis humaines et expérimentales à *Schistosoma mansoni, S. haematobium* et *S. japonicum*. *Ann. Parasit. hum. comp.*, **41**, 123.

Capron, A., Biguet, J., Vernes, A. and Afchain, D. (1968).   Structure antigenique des helminthes. Aspects immunologiques des relations hôte-parasite. *Path. Biol.*, **16**, 121.

Damian, R. T. (1967).   Common antigens between adult *Schistosoma mansoni* and the laboratory mouse. *J. Parasit.*, **53**, 60.

Grabar, P. and Burtin, P. (1964).   Immuno-electrophoretic Analysis. Elsevier Publishing Company.

Kagan, I. G. (1958).   Contributions to the immunology and serology of schistosomiasis. *Rice Inst. Pamph.*, **45**, 151.

Kagan, I. G. and Norman, L. (1963).   Analysis of helminth antigens. (*Echinococcus granulosus* and *Schistosoma mansoni*) *Ann. N.Y. Acad. Sci.*, **113**, 130.

Kent, N. H. (1963).   Comparative immunochemistry of larval and adult forms of *Schistosoma mansoni*. *Ann. N.Y. Acad. Sci.*, **113**, 100.

Smithers, S. R. and Terry, R. J. (1969).   The immunology of schistosomiasis. *Advances in Parasitology.*, **7**, 41.

Tsuji, M. (1968).   Immunoelectrophoretic studies in Parasitology. (in Japanese) *Igaku no ayumi.*, **67**, 531

Tsuji, M. (1971).   Serological diagnosis for helminthic diseases. (in Japanese) *J. Clin. Sci.*, **7**, 241.

Tsuji, M., Yokogawa, M., Capron, A. and Biguet, J. (1967).   Studies on the comparison of antigenic structure of three species of *Paragonimus* (*P. westermani, P. miyazakii* and *P. ohirai*). (in Japanese) *Jap. J. Parasit.* **16**, (*Suppl.*), 541.

Tsuji, M., Yokogawa, M. and Capron, A. (1968). Studies on precipitins of experimental infection with various species of *Paragonimus* in immunoelectrophoresis. (in Japanese) *Jap. J. Parasit.*, **17**, 596.

Tsuji, M., Yokogawa, M. and Capron, A. (1969). Studies on host-parasite relationship and antigenic communities between host and parasite by means of immunoelectrophoresis (I). (in Japanese) *Jap. J. Parasit.*, **18**, 387.

Yokogawa, M., Tsuji, M., Sano, M., Kojima, S. and Iijima, T. (1968). Studies on the immunological tests for schistosomiasis as the method of criterion of cure. (in Japanese) *Jap. J. Parasit.*, **17**, 288.

Complement Fixation and Hemagglutination Tests with Fractionated Antigens on Schistosomiasis

T. Sawada,* K. Takei,* K. Sato* and S. Sato**

*Department of Parasitology, School of Medicine, Gunma University,
Maebashi, Japan
**Department of Medical Zoology, School of Medicine,
Nagoya City University, Nagoya, Japan

INTRODUCTION

Fraction SPA prepared from lyophilized adult worms of *Schistosoma japonicum* by defatting, sonication, treatment with acetic acid and gel filtration on sephadex G100 column were reported by Sato *et al.* (1969) to be very reactive and specific for *S. japonicum* infections in the complement fixation and hemagglutiation tests, respectively. As the SPA fraction contained 44.3mg of protein and 1.4mg of carbohydrate, further separation of fraction SPA was conducted by gel-filtration on Bio-gel A-15m column and gel-filrtation on sephadex G100 column to obtain a more purified antigen of specificity and reactivity. The present paper deals with the results obtained from complement fixation and hemagglutination tests with prepared antigens.

MATERIALS AND METHODS

Two grams of lyophilized *S. japonicum* adult worms were defatted with diethyl-ether at $-20°C$ for 5 days, powdered and added to 200ml of 0.02M phosphate buffer pH 7, incubated at 2°C for 1 hr, sonicated at 10KC, 3.1 to 3.2mA for 30 min, and centrifuged at 14,000rpm for 15 min to get 191ml of supernatant SSI. The supernatant SSI which contained 680mg of protein and 94.5mg of carbohydrate was adjusted to pH 4.7 with 1N acetic acid, incubated at 2°C for 1 hr, and centrifuged at 14,000rpm for 15 min to obtain 190ml of supernatant, containing 244.4mg of protein and 68.2mg of carbohydrate and a sediment. A hundred ml of 0.1M phosphate buffer,

[179]

Fig. 1   Fractionation of Antigens for Complement Fixation and Hemagglutination Tests from *S. japonicum* Adult Worms

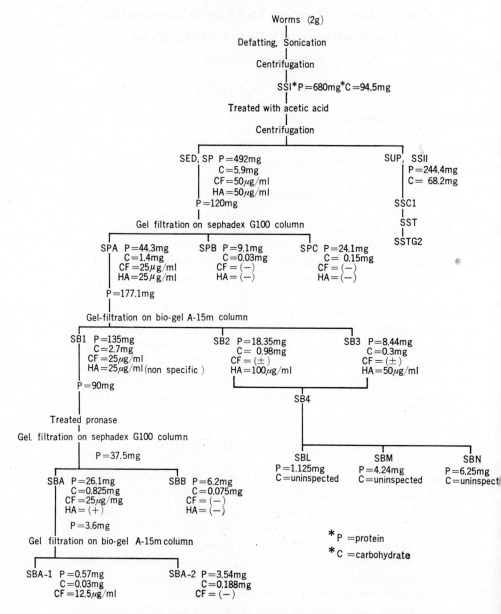

pH 8.0, was added to the sediment, which was them lyophilized to obtain antigen SP. Antigen SP contained 492mg protein and 5.9mg carbohydrate. Antigen SP was further fractionated as follows:

Gel-filtration by sephadex G 100

Sephadex G100 was washed repeatedly with distilled water, equilibrated with 0.05M phosphate buffer containing 0.05M NaCl, pH 7 and poured into a 2.0× 43 cm column. The column was charged with 10ml of SP fraction containing 120mg protein, and eluted with the same buffer at a flow rate of 25ml per hr, as shown in Fig. 2. Each 5ml of effluent was collected and analyzed for proteins and carbohydrates. Three fractions, SPA, SPB and SPC were obtained. Fraction SPA contained 44.3mg protein and 1.4mg carbohydrate; fraction SPB contained 9.1mg protein and 0.03mg carbohydrate; fraction SPC contained 24.1mg protein and 0.15mg carbohydrate.

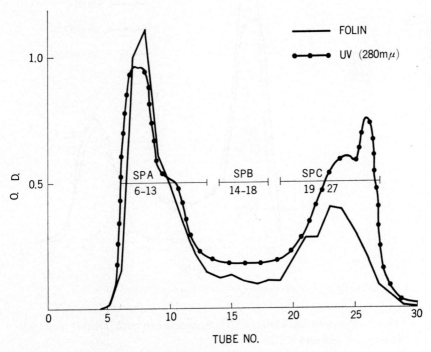

Fig. 2. Gel-Filtration on Sephadex G100 Column of Antigen SP

Gel-filtration on Bio-gel A-15m column

Fraction SPA was most reactive in the complement fixation test on schistosomiasis, and further purification of this antigen was attempted. Bio-gel A-15m column (2.0 × 43.0 cm) was prepared with 0.05M Tris and 0.001M ethyleneaminetetraacetic acid (EDTA) buffer, pH 7.6, containing 0.14M NaCl. The column was charged with 10ml of fraction SPA, containing 177.1mg of protein, and eluted with the same buffer at a flow rate of 25ml per hr, as shown in Fig. 3. Each 5ml of effluent was collected and analyzed for proteins and carbohydrates. Three fractions SB1, SB2 and SB3 were obtained. Fraction SB1 contained 135mg protein and 2.7mg carbohydrate; fraction SB2 contained 18.35mg protein and 0.98mg carbohydrate; fraction SB3 contained 8.44mg protein and 0.3mg carbohydrate.

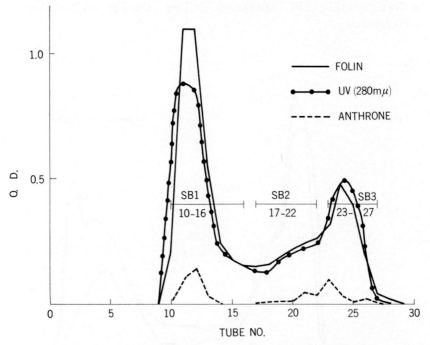

Fig. 3.   Gel-Filtration on Bio-Gel A-15m Column of Antigen SPA

Further separation of antigen SB1 by treatment with pronase and gel-filtration on sephadex G100 column

As fraction SB1 was most reactive, the further separation of this antigen was attempted. Nine hundred μg pronase and 2mg CaCl$_3$ were added to 6ml of fraction SB1 in 0.05M Tris-HCl buffer, pH 7.8, containing 90mg protein and kept at 37°C for 30 min. Sephadex G100 clumn (1.5 × 40 cm) was washed with deionized water. The column was charged with 2.5ml of fraction SB1 containing 37.5mg of protein, treated with pronase and eluted with deionized water at a flow rate of 20ml per hr, as shown in Fig. 4. Each 5ml of effluent was collected and analyzed for proteins and carbohydrates. Two fractions SBA and SBB were obtained. Fraction SBA contained 26.1mg protein and 0.825mg carbohydrate; fraction SBB contained 6.2mg protein and 0.075mg carbohydrate.

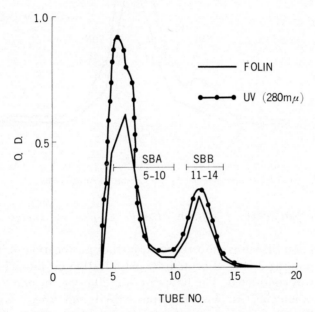

Fig. 4.   Gel-Filtration on Sephadex G100 Column of Antigen SPA Tested with Pronase

Further separation of fraction SB4

The fractions SB2 and SB3 were very reactive in the hemagglutination test. The fraction SB4, a mixture of SB2 and SB3, was separated by gel-filtration on Bio-gel A-15m column. Bio-gel A-15m column (1.0 × 40 cm) was prepared with 0.05M Tris and 0.001M EDTA buffer, pH 7.6, containing 0.14M NaCl. The column was charged with 6ml of fraction SB4, containing 15.22mg of protein, and eluted with the same buffer a flow rate of 20ml per hr, as shown in Fig. 5. Each 2.5ml of effluent was collected and analyzed for proteins and carbohydrates. Three fractions SBL, SBM and SBN were obtained. Fraction SBL contained 1.125mg protein; SBM contained 4.24mg protein; SBN contained 6.25mg protein. No carbohydrate was inspected from any of the 3 fractions.

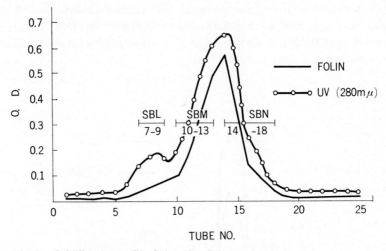

Fig. 5.   Gel-Filtration on Bio-Gel A-15m Column of Antigen SB4

Further purification of fraction SBA by gel-filtration Bio-gel A-15m column

As fraction SBA was most reactive, further purification of fraction SBA containing 3.6mg of protein by gel-filtration on Bio-gel A-15m column was conducted. The flow rate was 20ml per hr and 2.5ml of effluent was collected. Two fractions SBA-1 and SBA-2 were obtained (Fig. 6). Fraction SBA-1 contained 0.57mg protein and 0.03 mg carbohydrate; fraction SBA-2 contained 3.54mg protein and 0.188mg carbohydrate.

Complement fixation test: The test was conducted by the technique of Kimura (1964).

Hemagglutination test: The test was conducted by the technique of Lewis and Kessel (1961).

Analytical methods: Protein measurements were made with Folin reagent as described by Lowry *et al.* (1951). Carbohydrate measurements were made with Anthrone reagents (Morris, 1948).

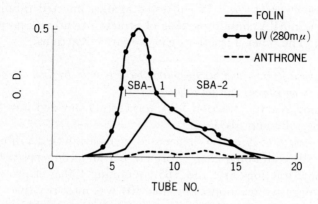

Fig. 6.   Gel Filtration on Bio-Gel A-15m Column of Antigen SBA

RESULTS

Complement fixation and hemagglutination tests with fractions SP and SSII
As fraction SSI was highly reactive, separation of this antigen into 2 fractions SP and SSII was carried out. Ten mg of each antigen was disolved in 10ml saline solution. The 1 : 1,000 saline solution was used as the solvent in these tests.

Complement fixation test: When tested against infected rabbit sera, the 2 fractions, SP containing $10\mu g$ of protein antigen per ml, and SSII containing $300\mu g$ of protein antigen per ml, gave reactions at dilutions of 1 : 8 and 1 : 1, respectively. When tested against infected human sera, the 2 fractions, SP containing $100\mu g$ of protein per ml, and SSII containing $145\mu g$ of protein per ml, gave reactions of 1 : 2 and 1 : 1, respectively.

Hemagglutination test: When tested against infected rabbit sera, the 2 fractions, SP containing $6.25\mu g$ of protein antigen per ml, and SSII containing $50\mu g$ of protein antigen per ml, gave reactions at dilutions of 1 : 200 and 1 : 800, respectively. When tested against infected human sera, only fraction SP containing $25\mu g$ of protein per ml was positive at a 1 : 800 dilution. Fraction SSII, containing $25\mu g$ of protein, gave a negative reaction.

Complement fixation and hemagglutination tests with fractions prepared by gel-filtration on sephadex G100 column
The highly reactive fraction SP was further separated into the 3 fractions SPA, SPB and SPC.

Complement fixation test: When tested against infected rabbit sera, only fraction SPA containing 25μg of protein per ml was positive in both test. The other 2 fractions gave negative reactions.

Complement fixation and hemagglutination tests with fractions prepared by gel-filtration on Bio-gel A-15m column

The most reactive fraction SPA was further devided into 3 fractions, SB1, SB2 and SB3.

Complement fixation test: When tested against infected rabbit sera, fraction SB1 containing 25μg of protein per ml gave a positive reaction. The 2 fractions SB2 and SB3 containing 100μg of protein per ml gave negative reactions. Fraction SB1 was most reactive.

Hemagglutination test: When tested against infected rabbit sera, the 2 fractions SB2 and SB3, each containing $100–50\mu$g of protein per ml, gave positive reactions. Fraction SB1, containing 25μg of protein per ml, gave a nonspecific reaction.

Complement fixation test prepared by gel-filtration on sephadex G100 column

The most reactive fraction SB1 for complement fixation test was further separated into 2 fractions, SBA and SBB.

Complement fixation test: When tested against infected rabbit sera, fraction SBA, containing 25μg of protein per ml, gave a positive reaction. Fraction SBB gave a negative reaction.

Complement fixation test prepared by gel-filtration on Bio-gel A-15m column

The highly reactive fraction SBA was further separated into 2 fraction, SBA-1 and SBA-2.

Complement fixation test: When tested against infected rabbit sera, fraction SBA-1, containing $6.25–12.5\mu$g of protein per ml, gave a positive reaction. Fraction SBA-2 gave a negative reaction.

Hemagglutination test prepared by gel-filtration on Bio-gel A-15m column

As fractions SB2 and SB3 were very reactive, the mixture SB4 of SB2 and SB3 was further divided into 3 fractions, SBL, SBM and SBN.

Hemagglutination test: When tested against infected rabbit sera, fraction SBL containing $12.5–25\mu$g of protein per ml, and fraction SBM containing $50–100\mu$g of protein per ml gave positive reactions.

Fraction SBN gave a negative reaction. Fraction SBL was most reactive.

SUMMARY

With antigens fractionated by gel-filtration on Bio-gel A-15m column and gel-filtration on sephadex G100, etc., complement fixation and hemagglutination tests were conducted and the following results were obtained:

1. Three fractions, SB1, SB2, and SB3, were obtained by gel-filtration on Bio-gel A-15m column from fraction SPA. Fraction SB1 was very reactive in complement fixation and hemagglutination tests but nonspecific in the hemagglutination test. Fractions SB2 and SB3 were reactive in the hemagglutination test.

2. Fractions SBA and SBB were obtained by digestion with pronase and gel-filtration on sephadex G100 column from SB1. Fraction SBA was very reactive in the complement fixation test and less reactive in hemagglutination test which might be due to the destrucruction of the antigenic substance by pronase.

3. Fractions SBA-1 and SBA-2 were obtained by gel-filtration on Bio-gel A-15m column from SBA. Fraction SBA-1 was most reactive in the complement fixation test. Fraction SBA-2 gave a negative reaction in complement fixation test.

4. Fraction SB4, a mixture of SB2 and SB3, was fractionated into 3 fractions, SBL, SBM and SBN, by gel-filtration on Bio-gel A-15m column. Fraction SBL was most reactive in hemagglutination test.

REFERENCES

Kimura, I. (1964). Methods in serology. X. Complement fixation test, *Protein Nucleic Acid Enzym.*, **9**, 663. (in Japanese)

Lewis, W. P. and Kessel, J. F. (1961). Hemagglutination in the diagnosis of toxoplasmosis and amebiasis. *Arch. Ophtal.*, **66**, 471.

Lowry, C. H., Rosebraugh, N. J., Farr, A. L. and Randall, R. J. (1951). Protein measurement with the Folin phenol reagent. *J. Biol. Chem.*, **193**, 265.

Morris, D. L. (1948). Quantitative determination of carbohydrates with Dreywood's anthrone reagent. *Science*, **107**, 254.

Sato, S., Sawada, T. and Takei, K. (1969). Studies on Complement Fixation and Hemagglutination Tests with Purified Antigens, SPA and SSCD2 in Infections with *Schistosoma japonicum*. *Japn. J. Exp. Med.*, **39**, 355.

Further Purification of *Schistosoma* Antigen
SSTG-2 by Gelfiltration on Sephadex G-100

T. SAWADA,* K. SATO,* K. TAKEI* and S. SATO**

*Department of Parasitology, School of Medicine, Gunma University,
Maebashi, Japan
**Department of Medical Zoology, School of Medicine,
Nagoya City University, Nagoya, Japan

INTRODUCTION

A purified skin test antigen SST was prepared by Williams *et al.* (1965) and Sawada *et al.* (1968) from lyophilized adult worms of *Schistosoma japonicum* by defatting with diethylether, sonic vibration, treatment with acetic acid, gel-filtration on sephadex G100 column, carboxymethyl (CM) cellulose column chromatography and diethylaminoethyl (DEAE) sephadex A50 column chromatography. Antigen SST was very reactive and the positive rate was 90.1% in the tests on 71 schistosomiasis patients. Control tests were performed on 62 "healthy" individuals. Of these, 30 were clonorchiasis patients who gave 3.2% false positive reactions. The antigen SST contained 4,060μg of protein and 87.5μg of carbohydrate per ml and was considered to be composed of several components with different molecular sizes and pI values which were mostly found in pH regions 4.0–6.0 by isoelectric focusing. Therefore, further separation by gel-filtration on sephadex G200 column was conducted to obtain SSTG-1 and SSTG-2 (Sawada *et al.*, 1969). In antigen SSTG-2, which was considered to be less than 200,000 in molecular weight and was most reactive on positive individuals with antigen SST, were found several proteins by disc electrophoresis (Sawada *et al.*, 1969).

Skin tests with antigen SSTG-2 on schistosomiasis patients and further separation of the antigen SSTG-2 were then attempted in order to study the substance responsible for the skin reaction.

[189]

MATERIALS AND METHODS

Preparation of antigen SSTG-1 and SSTG-2

Antigen SSTG-1 and SSTG-2 were prepared by the method described by Williams *et al.* (1965) and Sawada *et al.* (1968, 1969) (Fig. 1).

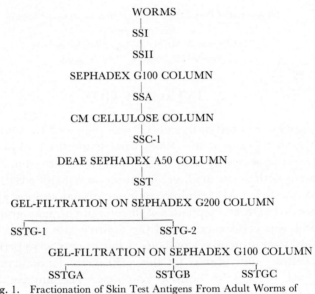

Fig. 1. Fractionation of Skin Test Antigens From Adult Worms of *Schistosoma japonicum*

Ultracentrifugal experiments with SSTG-2

An ultracentrifugal experiment with SSTG-2 was performed with a rotor speed of 59,780 rpm by the spinco model E ultracentrifuge. Before ultracentrifugation, SSTG-2 was dialyzed for 15 hrs against a solution of 0.02M phosphate buffer (P.B.), pH 6.0 and diluted with the same buffer to a final protein concentration of 1%. The sedimentation data were corrected to standard condition (s_{20}, w).

Gel-filtration on sephadex G100 column

As fraction SSTG-2 was most reactive and contained 2 peaks by ultracentrifugal analysis, further purification by gel-filtration on sephadex G100 column was attempted in order to study the substance responsible for the skin reaction. Sephadex G100 was washed repeatedly with 0.02M phosphate buffer, pH 6.0 and poured into a 1.2 × 45 cm column and equilibrated. The column was charged with

2.4 ml of fraction SSTG-2, containing 11.5 mg of protein, and eluted with 0.02M phosphate buffer, pH 6.0 at a flow rate of 8 ml per hr. Each 2 ml of effluent was collected and analyzed for proteins. Three fractions, SSTGA, SSTGB and SSTGC, were obtained (Fig. 1).

Disc electrophoresis

Disc electrophoresis was carried out by the method reported by Ornstein (1964) and Davis (1964) to study the proteins contained in fractions SSTG-2, SSTGA, SSTGB and SSTGC. Protein bands were detected by staining with amide black 10B.

Technique of skin testing

A half ml of 1:10,000 merthiolated saline was added to 10μg of each antigen, kept for 1 hr at room temperature, and then 1.5 ml of saline was added to it, so that 5 μg of antigen were contained in one ml. In making the skin tests, 0.02 ml of each antigen were injected intradermally into the volar surface of the forearm. The 0.1 μg of antigenic substance injected was estimated on the basis of total protein determined for each antigen. The mean diameter of the wheal appearing 15 min after the injection was measured. The positive reaction was $\geq$ 7 mm in mean diameter. The 0.2 μg of antigenic substance in 0.02 ml saline were injected into children (under 13 years old) who showed negative reactions by the injection of 0.1 μg of antigenic substance.

Analytical methods

The protein concentration of each antigen was determined by the method described by Lowry *et al.* (1951) with crystalline bovine serum albumin as the standard protein. The carbohydrate concentration was also determined by a method using anthrone reagent, with glucose as the standard carbohydrate.

RESULTS

Skin testing of antigens prepared by gel-filtration on sephadex G200 column chromatography of antigen SST

The 2 antigens SSTG-1 and SSTG-2 were tested at the 0.1 μg level on 22 patients (over 14 years old) infected with *S. japonicum* in Palo, Philippines. Antigen SSTG-2 was most reactive. Wheals over 7 mm diameter appeared within 5 to 15 min in all 22 individuals (100%) and gradually disappeared in size disappearing altogether within 1 hr.

Twenty-two proven schistosomiasis cases (over 14 years old) were also tested with 0.1 μg doses of SSTG-1. The reactions produced were of lesser intensity (36.4%) than those produced by SSTG-2 (Table 1).

Table 1. Skin Tests with Antigens SST, SSTG-1 and SSTG-2 on Individuals in Leyte, Philippines

Status		No. Tested	Antigen			
			Protein Content (μg/0.02ml)	SST	SSTG-1	SSTG-2
Patient*	Adult	22	0.1	15 (68.2)	8 (36.4)	22 (100)
	Child	31	0.1	0	—	13 (41.9)
	Child	23	0.2	—	—	21 (91.3)
Healthy	Adult	12	0.1	0	0	0
Control	Child	12	0.2	0	—	0

* Patient who demonstrated *Schistosoma japonicum* eggs in the stool.

Thirty-one children (under 13 years old) infected with *S. japonicum* were tested with 0.1 μg dose of SSTG-2 and positive reactions (wheals, 7.0 mm) appeared in 13 cases (41.9%). With injections of 0.1 μg doses of SSTG-1 into the 31 children, no positive reactions appeared.

As 0.1 μg dose of SSTG-2 was less reactive in the skin tests on children with schistosomiasis, 23 children infected with *S. japonicum* were tested with 0.2 μg doses of SSTG-2. Positive reactions were obtained in 21 cases (91.3%).

Both SSTG-1 and SSTG-2 gave negative reactions in 12 healthy individuals in doses of 0.1 and 0.2 μg.

Ultracentrifugal studies of SSTG-2

The physicochemical properties of SSTG-2 were studied by ultra-centrifugation. In Fig. 2, the sedimentation pattern of SSTG-2, taken 82 min after the rotor speed (59,780 rev./min.) had attained its maximum, is shown. Two main peaks appeared in it. The $s_{20}w$ value of peak I calculated from the ultracentrifugation data was 3.84, and that of peak II was 2.39. Those facts showed that 2 groups of proteins, with different molecular sizes, were present in SSTG-2.

Fractionation of SSTG-2 by gel-filtration technique

As SSTG-2 was most reactive, the further purification of this

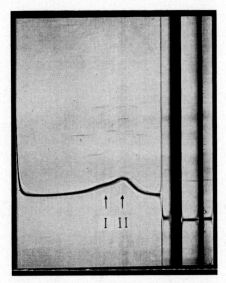

Fig. 2.   Sedimentation Pattern of Antigen SSTG-2 Exposure Taken after 82 Minutes.
   Rotor Speed was 59780 Rev./Min.

antigen was attempted. As SSTG-2 contained 2 groups of proteins, comparative experiments of separating it into 2 fractions by gel-filtration on each of sephadex G75, G100 G150 were attempted.
Three patterns were obtained (Fig. 3). Separation by gel-filtration on sephadex G100 was most satisfactory, as SSTG-2 was fractionated into 2 major peaks and one minor peak. Then 11.5 mg of SSTG-2 containing 744 μg of carbohydrate was fractionated by gel-filtration on sephadex G100 to obtain 3 fractions, SSTGA, SSTGB and SSTG-C, (Fig. 4) and the 3 fractions were concentrated by ultrafiltration using cellulose tubing, 8/32. Finally, 4.9 mg of SSTGA containing 374 μg of carbohydrate, 4.7 mg of SSTGB containing 70 μg of carbohydrate and 0.52 mg of SSTGC containing about 18 μg of carbohydrate were obtained.

Disc electrophoresis of antigens
   SSTGA, SSTGB and SSTGC were analyzed using 7% polyacrylamide gel to determine the components in these antigens (Fig. 5). By staining with amido black 10B, 3 protein bands with tailing were detected in SSTGA, 2 main protein bands with tailing and a minor

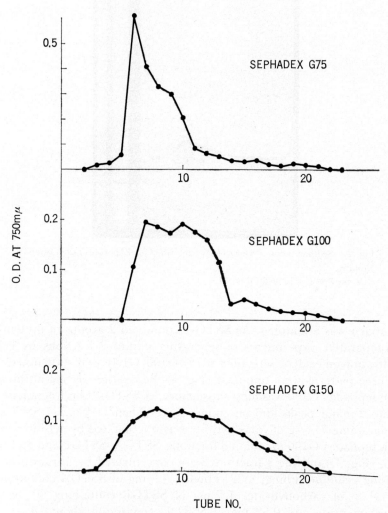

Fig. 3. Gel Filtration of SSTG-2 on Sephadex G75, G100 and G150
Column Size: 1.2×45 cm
Column Loading: 6.1 mg of Protein
Fraction Volume: 2 ml
Effluent Buffer: 0.02м P.B., pH 6.0
Flow Rate: 8 ml/hr.

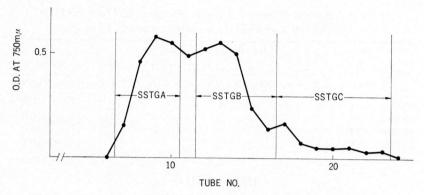

Fig. 4.   Fractionation of SSTG-2 by Gel-Filtration on Sephadex G100

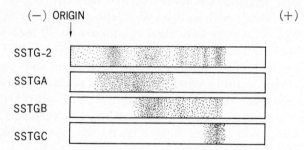

Fig. 5.   Disc Electrophoresis of Fractionated Antigens from SSTG-2

protein band were detected in SSTGB. SSTGC was composed of a
single protein band with tailing.

*Skin testing of antigens prepared by gel-filtration on sephadex G100 column
of antigen SSTG-2*

The 3 antigens SSTGA, SSTGB and SSTGC prepared from antigen SSTG-2 were tested at 0.1 μg level on 13 individuals infected
with *S. japonicum* in Yamanashi Prefecture, Japan (Table 2). Antigen
SSTGA was most reactive. Wheals 7 to 10.9 mm in diameter appeared in all 13 cases (100%). Antigen SSTGB was reactive. Wheals
7 to 10.9 mm in diameter appeared in 11 cases (84.6%). Antigen
SSTGC was also reactive and wheals 7 to 13.5 mm in diameter
appeared in 12 cases (92.3%). The three antigens SSTA, SSTB and
SSTC gave negative reactions in the tests on healthy individuals.

Table 2.   Results of Skin Tests with Antigens SSTG-2, SSTGA, SSTGB and SSTGC on Schistosomiasis Patients

Antigen	No. Tested	Mean diameter of wheal									No. Positive	% Positive
		0–5.9	6–6.9	7–7.9	8–8.9	9–9.9	10–10.9	11–11.9	22–12.9	13–UP		
SSTG-2	13			4	2	3	2	1	1		13	100.0
SSTGA	13			6	2	4	1				13	100.0
SSTGB	13		2	7	1	1	2				11	84.6
SSTGC	13		1	6	2	2		1		1	12	92.3

DISCUSSION

In paper mentioned above (Sawada *et al.*, 1969), it was reported that antigen SSTG-2 was more reactive than antigen SSTG-1 on positive individuals with antigen SST, the positive rate of SSTG-2 being 100%. Skin tests were then conducted on 22 individuals infected with *S. japonicum* with the 3 antigens SSTG-1, SSTG-2 and SST. Antigen SSTG-1 produced positive reactions in 8 cases (positive rate, 36.4%), antigen SSTG-2 provoked positive reactions in all 22 cases (positive rate, 100%) and antigen SST provoked positive reactions in 15 cases (positive rate, 68.2%). Accordingly, antigen SSTG-2 was a most reliable antigen for the diagnosis of schistosomiasis japonica.

The three antigens, SSTGA, SSTGB and SSTGC were separated from antigen SSTG-2 by gel-filtration. These antigens were similar to the 3 antigens, SSTA1 SSTA2 and SSTA3 prepared from antigen SST by disc-sephadex G25 column electrophoresis and disc electrophoresis described by Sato *et al.* (1969). SSTGA contained common protein in SSTA1. SSTGB contained common protein in SSTA1 and SSTA2. SSTGC was similar to SSTA3. There was no significant difference between the positive rates obtained statistically by injection with the 3 antigens SSTGA, SSTGB and SSTGC. Antigen SSTA1, SSTA2 and SSTA3 were all reactive in the skin test. From these results, it was considered that almost all proteins in SSTG-2 provoked positive reactions.

By injection of antigen SSTG-2 into 31 children infected with *S. japonicum* in doses of 0.1 μg, positive reactions appeared in 13 cases (41.9%). By injection of antigen SSTG-2 (0.2 μg) into 23 cases infected with *S. japonicum*, positive reactions appeared in 21 cases (91.3%). These facts may suggest that the antibody titer in children is lower than in adults, due to the difference in activity of antibody production against *S. japonicum* in children and in adults, or because of the stage of infection. However, the possibility that chemical reaction such as histamine release may be different in children cannot be excluded.

SUMMARY

1. Antigen SSTG-2 prepared from antigen SST was most reactive in schistosomiasis patients, the detection rate being 100%.

2. Antigens SSTGA, SSTGB and SSTGC were prepared from purified antigen SSTG-2 by gel-filtration on sephadex G100 column. The 3 antigens were all reactive in the skin tests on 13 schistosomiasis patients in doses of 0.1 μg, positive rates of SSTGA, SSTGB and SSTGC being 100%, 84.6% and 92.3%, respectively.

3. Antigens SSTGA and SSTGB each contained 3 proteins. SSTGC contained a single protein.

REFERENCES

Davis, B. J. (1964).   Disc electrophoresis. II. Method and application to human serum protein. *Ann. N.Y. Acad. Sci.*, **121**, 404.

Lowry, O. H., Rosebrough, N. J., Farr, A. L. and Randall, R. J. (1951).   Protein measurement with Folin phenol reagent. *J. Biol. Chem.*, **193**, 265.

Ornstein, L. (1964).   Disc electrophoresis. I. Background and theory. *Ann. N.Y. Acad. Sci.*, **121**, 321.

Sato, K., Sawada, S. and Sato, S. (1969).   Studies on the Purification of Skin Test Antigen SST for the Diagnosis of schistosomiasis japonica. II. The Purification of Antigen SST by Disc-Sephadex G25 Column Electrophoresis and Disc Electrophoresis. *Jap. J. Exp. Med.*, **39**, 347.

Sawada, T., Sato, S., Takei, K., Moose, J. W. and Williams, J. E. (1968).   Immunodiagnosis of schistosomiasis. III. Further purification of antigen SSC1 by DEAE sephadex A50 column chromatography. *Exp. Parasitology*, **23**, 238.

Sawada, T., Sato, K. and Sato, S. (1969).   Studies on the Purification of Skin Test Antigen SST for the Diagnosis of schistosomiasis japonica. I. The Characterization and Purification of antigen SST by Zone Electrophoresis and Gel-filtration Technique. *Jap. J. Exp. Med.*, **39**, 339.

Williams, J. E., Moose, J. W., Sawada, T., Takei, K. and Sato, S. (1965).   Studies on the immunodiagnosis of schistosomiasis. I. Intradermal skin tests with fractionated antigens. *J. Inf. Dis.*, **115**, 382.

Ultrastructural Observation of the Circumoval Precipitation of *Schistosoma japonicum*

D. Sakumoto,* Y. Tongu,* S. Suguri,* D. Itano,*
S. Inatomi,* H. Tanaka** and H. Matsuda**

*Department of Parasitology, Okayama University Medical School,
Okayama, Japan
**Department of Parasitology, Institute of Medical Science,
University of Tokyo, Tokyo, Japan

I. INTRODUCTION

The circumoval precipitation test reported by Oliver-Gonzalez (1954), is an immuno-serological reaction which induces precipitation around the schistosome egg when the egg is soaked in the antiserum of this parasite. This immunodiagnosis method for schistosomiasis has since become a very important one for many researchers.

Circumoval precipitation appears globular or club-shaped with vacuole or oil droplet-like substances around the outer surface of the egg shell. Under the light microscope it is observed just as it stream out of the egg shell.

This paper deals with observation on the ultrastructure of the circumoval precipitation of *Schistosoma japonicum*.

II. MATERIALS AND METHODS

Circumoval precipitation was produced by placing 0.3 cc of antiserum and 0.3 cc egg suspension of *S. japonicum* togeth with salines solution and 0.06 cc marsonin solution (1:1000) in reagent glass, and then incubating at 37°C for 24 hours in a vacuum incubator. The eggs with circumoval precipitation were collected from the reagent glass and fixed with 2% glutaraldehyde solution for half an hour, and post-fixed with 1% osmium tetroxide solution for 12 hours. The eggs were dehydrated in ethanol and embedded in Epon. Sections were cut with a Porter-Blum Ultramicrotome and were placed on copper coated grids and double stained with uranyl acetate and lead nitrate. These specimens were observed with a Hitachi HS-8 electron microscope.

III. RESULTS

a. Normal egg

The thickness of the egg shell of *Schistosoma japonicum* is about 0.68 μ and on the outer surface are numerous densely growing micro-villi-like projections. Each projection is about 260 Å in diameter and about 1–2 μ in length. There are about 900 such projections in one square micron of the egg shell surface. Numerous irregularly formed, densely packed granules, each less than 750 Å in diameter, were found in the egg shell layer, but no other structure was found (Figs. 1 and 2).

b. Egg treated with antiserum

When *Schistosoma* eggs were placed in antiserum, precipitation in the form of globules, as observed under the light microscope appeared around the outer surface of the egg shell (Fig. 3). These globules varied in size and shape, and were sometimes elongate.

In the early positive stage of the circumoval precipitation under the electron microscope, a small clot or thin layered precipitation appeared on the brush-like projections of the outer surface of the egg shell (Fig. 4). The precipitation clot grew thicker and larger, and covered the egg shell surface. It could not be seen under the light microscope until this stage of precipitation (Fig. 5). The precipitation clot was composed of fine grains and fine fibril networks (Type A precipitation). The eruption of the large precipitation clot from the egg shell surface had the appearance of volcano smoke or oil droplet-like globules (Figs. 6, 7, and 8). The elongate granules observed under the light microscope were highly dense and varied in size and shape (Type B precipitation), and were surrounded with thick layers of the A-type precipitation (Fig. 9). The microvilli-like projections or the fragments of those were observed in the clot in some cases (Fig. 8). Some large globular circumoval precipitations contain several vacuolar circumoval precipitation clots (Figs. 12 and 13).

Usually the large, vacuolar, precipitation clot appears at the weak point on the egg shell, such as the thinner portion of the egg shell (Fig. 10) or at a point of breakage by mechanical means. A cir-cumoval precipitation clot erupts from these parts around the center of the clot, and a precipitation clot of the same structure appears at the same place inside the egg shell (Figs. 11, 12, and 13). No limiting membrane could be found around the circumoval precipitation clot.

IV. DISCUSSION

Inatomi (1962), Inatomi *et al.* (1970) and Hockley (1968) described the ultrastructure of *Schistosoma* eggs. These egg shells are of an extremely complicated structure, having numerous microvilli-like projections on the egg shell surface and a small number of very fine canals in the amorphous egg shell matrix. This structure served a significant role in the circumoval precipitation test. It is supposed that the metabolic product streams out of the fine canals of the egg shell, while the antiserum products infiltrate the inside of the egg shell. The microvilli-like projections are believed to be a relevant element in this phenomenon. In either case, at the outer surface of the egg shell, the antiserum and the metabolic products combine to produce the circumoval precipitation. The extent of the circumoval precipitation is determined by the extent and dimensions of the streaming of the embryo's metabolic products out of the egg shell canals.

SUMMARY

The circumoval precipitation of *S. japonicum* was observed with the electron microscope. No limiting or border line at the outer surface of the circumoval precipitation clot can be seen with the electron microscope. It is very difficult to observe the thin layered circumoval precipitation clot, which is less than 1 μ thick. Circumoval precipitation appears not only on the outer surface of the egg shell but also in the inner space between the egg shell and embryo.

A and B type precipitation are found in the precipitation clot. A type is composed of fine grains and a fine fibril network, and B type is highly dense, irregular in size and composed of large granules. The circumoval precipitation clot is found very often at the defective portion of the egg shell.

REFERENCES

Inatomi, S. (1962). Submicroscopic structure of the egg shell of helminth. *Okayama Igakkai Zasshi*, **74** (1–3) Supp., 31.

Inatomi, S., Tongu, Y., Sakumoto, D., Suguri, S., and Itano, K. (1970). Ultrastructure of *Schistosoma japonicum*. Recent Advances in Researches on Filariasis and Schistosomiasis in Japan. Univ. Tokyo Press, 257.

Kemp, W. M. (1970). Ultrastructure of the cercarienhullen reaction of *Schistosoma mansoni*. *J. Parasit.*, **56**(4), 713.

Oliver-Gonzalez, J. (1954). Anti-egg precipitins in the serum of humans infected with *Schistosoma mansoni*. *J. Infect. Dis.*, **96**, 86.

Oliver-Gonzalez, J. (1955). Species specificity of the anti-egg precipitin in *Schistosoma serum*. *J. infect. Dis.*, **96**, 95.

Yokogawa, M., Sano, M., and Araki, K. (1967). Immunosero-diagnosis of Schistosomiasis japonica. 3. Circumoval precipitation test. *Jap. J. Parasit.*, **16**(2), 77.

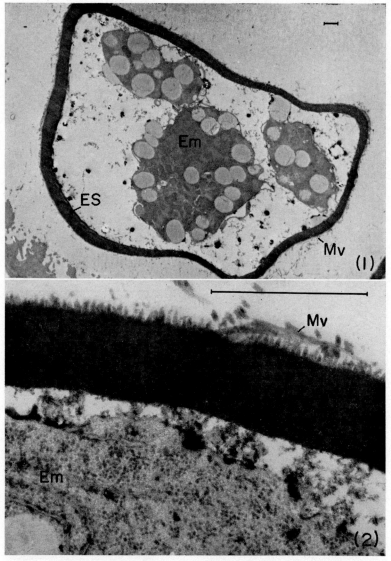

Fig. 1.   Egg of *Schistosoma japonicum*.
Fig. 2.   Microvilli Distributed on the Outer Surface of the Egg Shell.
   There are fragments of the embryo inside the egg shell.
   COP; circumoval precipitation, Em; embryo, ES; egg shell, Mv; microvilli, P_1, P_2; precipitation.

(Scale is one micron in each micrograph)

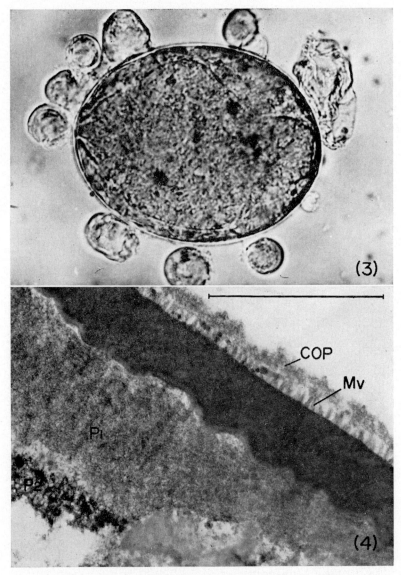

Fig. 3.   Egg with the Circumoval Precipitation.
   Circumoval precipitation is vacuole-like.
Fig. 4.   Egg Shell Surface with Extremely Positive Circumoval Precipitation.
Thin layered circumoval precipitation covers the microvilli layer. Inside of the
egg shell is seen fine granulated precipitation (P1) and irregularly formed,
highly dense precipitation (P2).

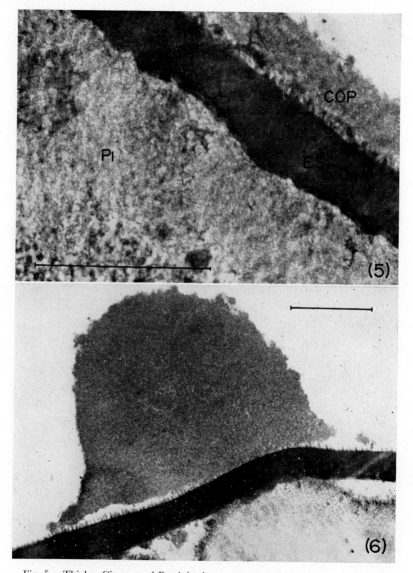

Fig. 5.   Thicker Circumoval Precipitation.
   Inside of the egg shell also seen circumoval precipitation.
Fig. 6.   Large Swollen Circumoval Precipitation Clot on the Egg Shell.

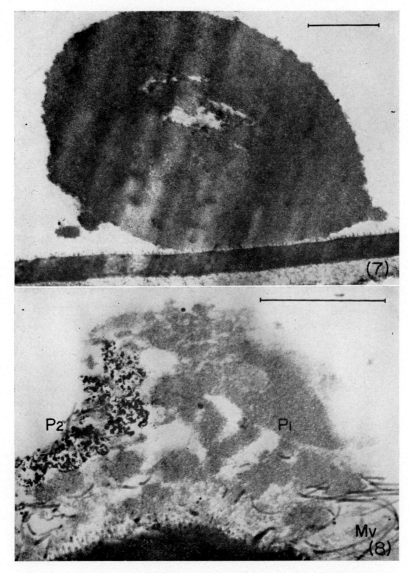

Fig. 7.   Oil Droplet Like Circumoval Precipitation Clot on the Egg Shell Surface.

Fig. 8.   Circumoval Precipitation Clot on the Egg Shell.

P1 Type precipitin with tangling microvilli and P2 Type precipitin are seen.

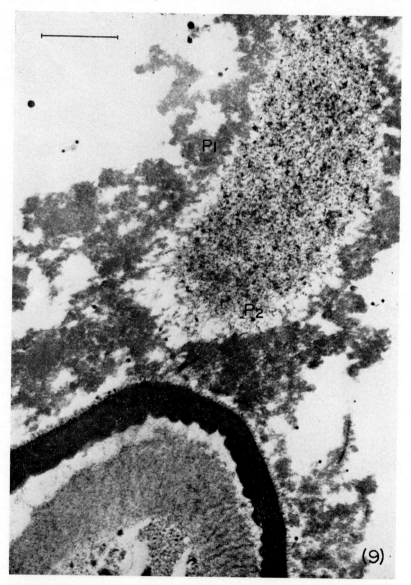

Fig. 9. Large and Irregularly Formed Circumoval Precipitation Clot on the Egg Shell.

P2 Type precipitin is surrounded by P1 Type precipitin.

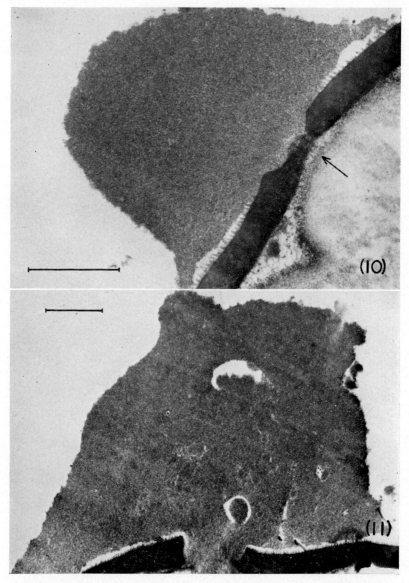

Fig. 10. Large Circumoval Precipitation Clot Extending above an Egg Shell Defect.

Fig. 11. Circumoval Precipitation Clot Flowing out of the Egg Shell Defect.

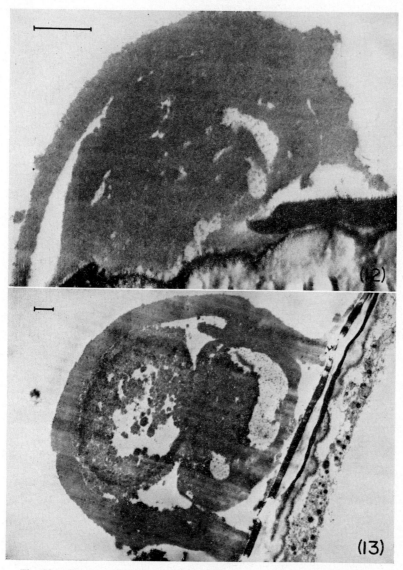

Fig. 12.   Circumoval Precipitation Clot Flowing out of the Egg Shell Defect.
Fig. 13.   Oil Droplet Like Circumoval Precipitation Clot Extending above of
the Egg Shell Defect.

Two circumoval precipitation clots are distinguished in it.

Ultrastructure of Cercaria of *Schistosoma spindale*

S. Inatomi, D. Sakumoto, Y. Tongu, S. Suguri,
K. Itano and T. Saito

*Department of Parasitology, Okayama University Medical School,
Okayama, Japan*

I. INTRODUCTION

Inatomi *et al.* (1970 a, b) studied the cercaria of *Schistosoma japonicum* through the electron microscope, and described the integument, muscle, excretory system, sense organ, secretory organ, and digestive organ. Especially, in helminths, the striated muscle cells arranged vertically in the tail of the cercaria showed a characteristic form in a cross section. Such morphological features common to all cercaria were reported.

Following the previous report, this paper reports on the ultrastructure of the cercaria of *Schistosoma spindale*.

II. MATERIALS AND METHODS

Cercariae of *Shistosoma spindale* collected for the study were those that escape naturally from the experimentally infected snail host, *Indoplanorbis exustus*. The cercariae were immediately fixed in cold 1% glutaraldehyde solution buffered with phosphate (pH 7.4) for 30 minutes, and then washed with phosphate buffer. They were post-fixed with cold 2% osmium tetroxide solution (pH 7.4) for 1 hour, dehydrated with an ethanol series by the routine methods and embedded in styrene methacrylate. Specimens were cut with Porter-Blum Ultramicrotome, and thin sections were stained with uranyl acetate and lead nitrate. A Hitachi HS-8 electron microscope was used for the observations.

III. RESULTS

1. *Integument*

The outer surface of the body and the tail of the cercaria is covered

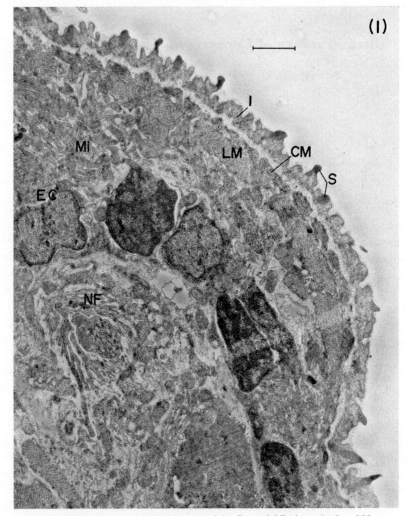

Fig. 1.   Cross Section of the Head Part of the Cercarial Body at the Level Near the Nerve Center.

The body surface is covered by the thin integumentary layer with small spines. The fiber layer and the muscle layer lie under the integumentary layer. The nerve ganglion is situated outside of the head muscle.

B. basement membrane, Ci. cilium, CM. circular muscle, D. desmosome, EC. epidermal cell, ExC. excretory canal, F. fiber layer, I. integument, LM. longitudinal muscle, M. muscle layer, Mi. mitochondria, Mv. microvillus, N. nucleus, NF. nerve fiber, P. plasma membrane, S. spine, SB. sensory bulb, SG. secretory granule, Tk. thick myofilament, Tn. thin myofilament.

(Scale is one micron in each micrograph)

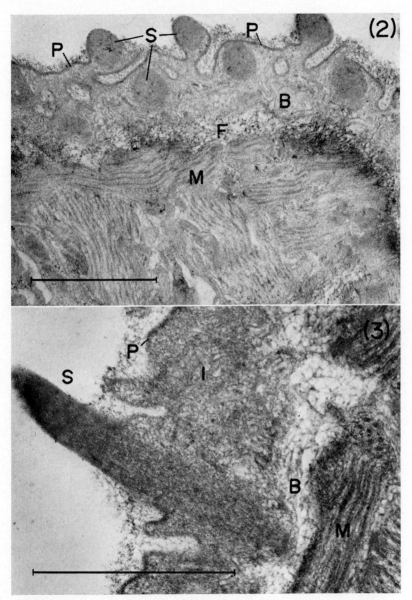

Fig. 2. Cross Section of the Integument.

The outside of the integument is covered with a thin plasma membrane. There can be seen small spines and a number of the infoldings of the basal plasma membrane in the matrix of the integumentary layer. The fiber layer which is constructed of the network of very thin fibers, and the muscle layer which has thick and thin myofilaments and belongs to the somatic muscle, can be observed under the integumentary layer.

Fig. 3. Longitudinal Section of the Spine.

The spine has a lattice-like crystaloid structure. The extruding part of the spine from the integumentary layer and the rootlet of the spine reach the basal plasma membrane of the integumentary layer.

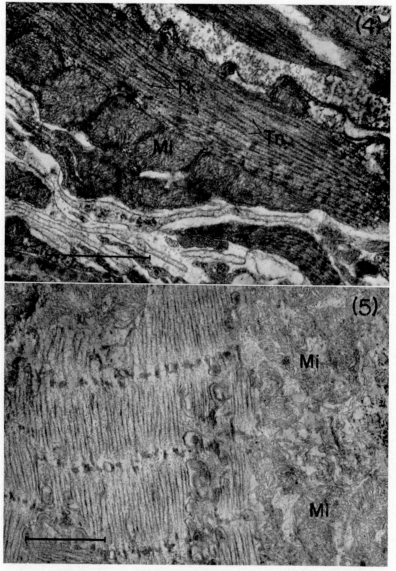

Fig. 4.   Longitudinal Section of a Body Muscle Fiber.
     There can be seen thick and thin myofilaments, and mitochondria with
many cristae.
Fig. 5.   Longitudinal Section of the Tail Longitudinal Striated Muscle.
     Thick and thin myofilaments and dense bodies, Z-discs can be seen, but the I
and the A bands are not apparent.

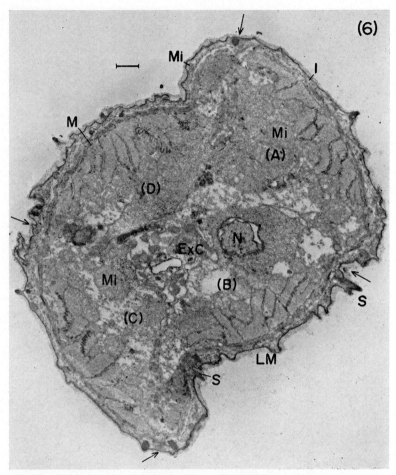

Fig. 6, 7.   Cross Section of the Tail at the Flame Cell Level.

The tail surface is covered with the thin integument and the circular muscle layer which consists of the smooth muscles located beneath the integumentary layer. The longitudinal muscle which is situated under the circular muscle layer is arranged regularly and divided into four muscle groups (A.B.C.D.), each group having 5 muscle cells.

The borders of the four muscle groups are indicated by four arrows.

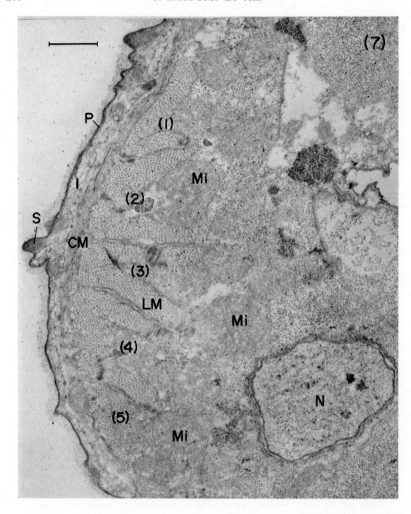

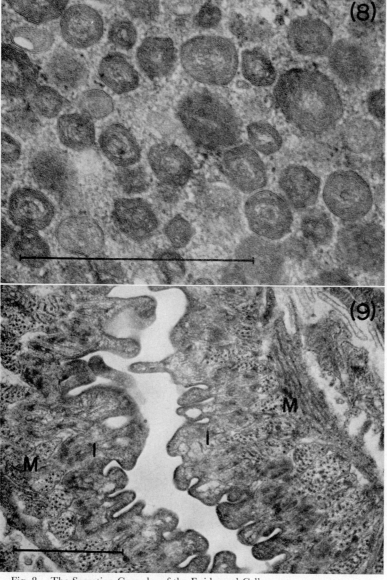

Fig. 8.   The Secretion Granules of the Epidermal Cell.
    The secretion granules have a lamellar structure.
Fig. 9.   Cross Section of the Oral Sucker.
    The luminal surface of the oral sucker is covered with the integumentary
layer which has infoldings of the basal plasma membrane. The muscle layer is
located beneath the integumentary layer.

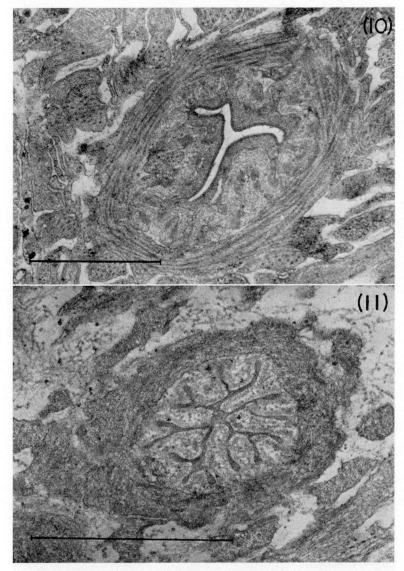

Fig. 10.   Cross Section of the Esophagus.
   The esophagus has the triradiate lumen which is covered with the thin integumentary layer, and surrounded by the circular muscle layer.
Fig. 11.   Cross Section of the Lower Part of the Esophagus.
   The esophageal lumen is branching in complicated.

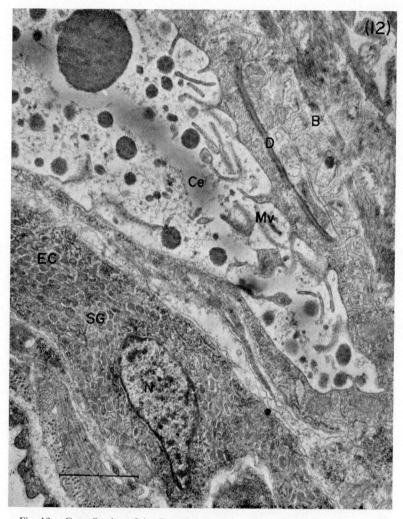

Fig. 12. Cross Section of the Cecum.

Small microvilli-like projections are distributed on the luminal surface of the cecum. Many infoldings of the basal plasma membrane, mitochondria and the desmosome are observable in the intestinal epithelial cell. The epidermal cell with many secretory granules can be seen at the lower part of the picture.

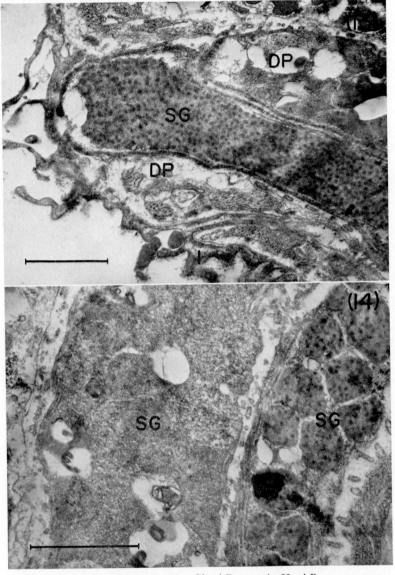

Fig. 13.   Opening of the Penetration Gland Duct at the Head Part.
Fig. 14.   The penetration gland duct is full of countless secretion granules.

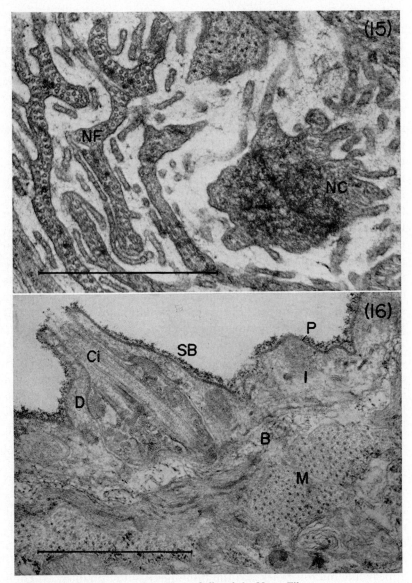

Fig. 15.   Cross Section of the Nerve Cell and the Nerve Fibers.
Each of them has many microtubules.
Fig. 16.   Longitudinal Section of the Sensory Bulb on the Body Integument.
The outside of the sensory bulb is covered with the integument. The sensory
bulb has a cilium connecting to the nerve fiber at the bottom of the sensory bulb.

with a thin integument, 0.1 to 0.5 μ in thickness. Like other trematodes, the integument is connected to epidermal cells, which lie under
the muscle layer in the deep portion of the body, by protoplasmic
tubules formed from plasma membrane. The integumentary layer
that covers the whole body surface together with a number of the
epidermal cells forms a large syncytium. Nuclei are visible in the
epidermal cells but not in the integumentary layer. Both the outer
surface and the basal surface of the integument are bordered by a
thin plasma membrane about 100 Å thick. In the matrix of the integument, there are numerous discoidal dense granules, vacuoles,
minute spines, mitochondria and infoldings of the basal plasma
membrane. Discoidal granules vary in size and have a concentric
lamellated structure. The granule surface is covered with a thin
membrane about 80 Å in thick. Several infoldings from the basal
plasma membrane into the matrix can be seen. A minute spine
presents a crystalloid lattice-like structure of 2 μ in length and 0.1 μ
in diameter. The spine part extending out of the integument is
covered with the same thin plasma membrane that covers the outer
surface of the integument. The rootlets of the spines reach the basal
plasma membrane of the integument.

2. *Fiber layer*

The fiber layer of the connective tissue, situated between the
integumentary layer and the muscle layer, is composed of a fine
fibril network made from collagen-like thin filaments. Each filament
is approximately 80 Å in diameter. The thin fiber layer is between
1/3 to 1/4 as thick as the integumentary layer.

3. *Body muscle*

Four groups are distinguished as the body muscle under the fiber
layer. They are circular, longitudinal, diagonal and dorso-ventral
muscles. These all belong to the somatic muscle which have two kinds
of the myofilaments, thick ones, about 250 Å in diameter, and thin
ones, about 50 Å in diameter. In cross section the thick myofilaments
appear like microtubules and the thin ones like the small spots. Each
thick myofilament is surrounded by about 12 thin myofilaments,
arranged hexagonally. A large number of mitochondria, glycogen
particles, nuclei, etc. are visible in the peripheral parts of the muscle
cells.

4. *Tail muscle*

The outer circular muscle layer and the inner longitudinal muscle layer can be seen in the tail. As in most of the trematode groups, the outer circular muscle layer belongs to the somatic muscle and the inner longitudinal muscle layer to the striated muscle. In the cross section of the tail at the flame cell level, the integument is visible as the outermost layer, followed by the outer circular muscle inside, and the inner longitudinal muscle and the excretory tubule in the center. Within these regions, the inner longitudinal muscle is divided into four groups of muscles, each including 4 to 5 striated muscle cells. Countless glycogen particles and mitochondria with many cristae are distributed between the myofibrils in each muscle cell. In longitudinal section, the dense Z discs of the myofibrils of the striated muscle are observable, but A and I bands are not.

5. *Epidermal cells*

The epidermal cells are situated under the muscle layer, and are connected with the integumentary layer by thin protoplasmic tubules. The cells, including the nuclei, are filled with an extensively ramifying Golgi complex and endoplasmic reticula with fine granules among which the mitochondria, glycogen particles, and lamellar dense discoidal granules of various sizes are distributed.

6. *Nervous system*

The nerve ganglion composed of bundles of microtubules is situated at the bottom of the head muscle on both lateral sides. These microtubules are approximately 100 Å in diameter and may be the nerve fibers. In several portions of the integument of body wall, sensory bulbs about 1μ in diameter can be distinguished, many of which appear to have only one cilium, and some with a few cilia. The sensory bulb is folded with the rootlets of the cilia protruding deeply into the desmosome, while the microtubules (or nerve fibers) appear to reach to the bottom of the sensory bulb. A dense body and mitochondria can be seen in the bulb.

7. *Digestive organ*

The integumentary layer about 1 to 2 μ in thickness forms a continuous surface layer over the inside of the oral sucker and duct. The oral sucker especially has an intensely convoluted surface from the

basal plasma membrane. The lumen at the upper part of the esophagus is triple-layered, and as it proceeds to the lower part of the
esophagus, the lumen forks repeatedly to make a branching complex. The end of the esophagus leads into the primitive structured
cecum. Thin microvilli-like projections, composed of very thin
epithelial cells from the inner layer of the cecal wall, protrude into
the lumen.

8. *Penetration glands*

There are five pairs of penetration glands on each lateral side of
the body. The structure is therefore similar to that of cercaria belonging to other schistosome groups. There are two kinds of penetration
glands, the anterior two pairs being distinctly different from the
posterior three pairs, which are characterized by the structure of the
granular particles in the gland cells. In the duct wall connected with
these gland cells, there are microtubules tightly packed in parallel
and arranged longitudinally.

9. *Excretory system*

The excretory system has almost the same structure as that of most
of the trematode groups. It begins with the flame cell which bears
more than 80 cilia. Some cilia and thin microvilli-like projections are
distributed on the way from the flame cell to the excretory tubules.

IV. DISCUSSION

Soparker (1921) gave a detailed account, based on light microscopy, of the morphology of *S. spindale* cercaria. As for the fine structure of the cercaria of trematode, Cardel and Philpott (1960) observed the tail of *Himasthla quissetensis* cercaria and indicated, "A
layer of smooth muscle, with its fibers running perpendicular to the
long axis of the tail lies internal to the cuticle. A layer of striated
muscle with the fibers directed spirally around the tail is located
beneath the smooth muscle." Inatomi *et al.* (1964) observed the
cercaria of *Clonorchis sinensis* and indicated that the striated muscle
layer of the tail is divided into four muscle groups, each group with a
definite number of the muscle cells. The distribution of muscle cells
in each muscle group is determined by the species of helminths.
Both in *S. japonicum* and *S. mansoni*, it is supposed that 4 to 5 striated

muscle cells belong to one of four muscle groups. Similarly, the muscle of *S. spindale* is divided into four groups, with 4 to 5 cells in each.

There are several reports on the body wall structure, Kruidenier and Vatter (1958) on *S. mansoni*, Lautenschlager and Cardell (1959) and Cardell (1962) on *H. quissetensis*, Belton and Harris (1967) on *Acanthatrium oregonensis*, Inatomi *et al.* (1970 a, b) on the cercaria of *S. japonicum*, and Tongu *et al.* (1970) on *Cercaria longissima*. These observations may be summarized jointly as follows: The integument varies in different regions of the body, and consists of three components, which are the outer thin plasma membrane, the middle thick matrix and the basal plasma membrane. Many vacuoles, vesicles with fibrillar contents, spines and several hairs are scattered in the integument. The cercarial integument is thinner than that of the adult. Hackley (1968) and Robson and Erasmus (1970) observed the cercaria of *Schistosoma mansoni* with the scanning electron microscope and reported that abundant projections and protrusions can be seen on the body wall surface.

Lumsden and Foor (1968) observed the body and tail muscles of the cercaria of *Heterobilharzia americana* and stated that there are striated myofibrils in the tail but there are no A and I bands as in other animals. Inatomi *et al.* (1970 a, b) made similar observations.

Dixon and Mercer (1965) stated that the sensory processes in cercaria of *Fasciola hepatica* function as a tangorecepter. Morris and Threadgold (1967) also observed the sensory organ in *S. mansoni*, and Rees (1967) the neuropile in *Parorchis acanthus*. The nervous system and the sensory organ observed by Halton and Morris (1969), Lyons (1969 a, b) and Wilson (1970), were reported in detail. In *S. spindale* some of the sensory organs contain sensory hairs with the nervepile and a cilium and some of them contain sensory hairs with more than two cilia. In spite of the varieties of structures, the sensory organ shows an identical structure to the peripheral apparatus of nervous system. Particularly many sensory organs can be seen at the tip of the head of the cercaria. Reissig (1970) reported on the axon in *S. mansoni*. The structure of the neuropile observed by Dixon and Mercer (1965) and Rees (1967) is remarkably similar in the two species.

The anatomical features which are common to all these species are also common to *S. spindale*.

SUMMARY

Cercaria of *S. spindale* were observed under the electron microscope. The integument is connected to the epidermal cells, and forms a large syncytium as other cercariae. Numerous discoidal, dense secretory granules, vacuoles, mitochondria, minute spines and infoldings of the basal plasma membrane are distributed in the matrix of the integument.

The secretory granules are limited by a thin membrane on the outer surface, and form a concentric lamella. The minute spines reveal crystalloid and lattice-like structure. The fine fibril network of the connective tissue is located between the integumentary and muscle layers. The cercarial body has circular, longitudinal, diagonal and dorso-ventral muscle layers. They belong to the somatic muscle which has thin and thick myofilaments. The cercarial tail has the outer, circular muscle which belongs to the somatic muscle. Four striated muscle groups are observed in cross section at the flame cell level of the tail. Each muscle group has four or five striated muscle cells as do other *Schistosoma* cercariae.

Epidermal cells located beneath the muscle layer are connected to each other and to the integument to form a syncytium. The excretory system is very simple and has several flame cells as the protonephridium. The nervous commissure including numerous nerve fibers can be observed at the lower part of the head apparatus on both sides. The sensory bulb with a cilium as the sense organ can be found in the integumentary layer.

Acknowledgements

We express our sincere appreciation to Dr. Lee Kian Joe of Institute of Medical Research, Kuala Lumpur, Malaysia, for his very kind help in providing *S. spindale* cercaria from his laboratory. Thanks are also due to the Japan-United States Cooperative Medical Science Program for their support toward this study.

REFERENCES

Belton, C. M. and Harris, P. J. (1967).   Fine structure of the cuticle of the cercaria of *Acanthatrium oregonensis* (Macy). *J. Parasit.*, **53**, 715.
Cardell, R. R. and Philpott, D. E. (1960).   The ultrastructure of the tail of the cercaria of *Himasthla quissentensis* (Miller and Northup, 1926) *Trans. Am. Micro. Soc.*, **79**, 442.

Cardell, R. R. (1962). Observations on the ultrastructure of the body of the cercaria of *Himasthla quissentensis* (Miller and Northup, 1926). *Trans. Am. Micro. Soc.*, **81**, 124.

Dixon, K. E. and Mercer, E. H. (1965). The fine structure of the nervous system of the cercaria of the liver fluke, *Fasciola hepatica* L. *J. Parasit.*, **51**, 967.

Hackley, D. J. (1968). Scanning electron microscopy of *Schistosoma mansoni* cercaria. *J. Parasit.*, **54**, 1241.

Halton, D. W. and Morris, G. P. (1969). Occurrence of cholinesterase and ciliated sensory structures in a fish gill-fluke, *Diclidophora merlangi* (Trematoda: Monogenea). *Z. Parasitenk.*, **33**, 21.

Inatomi, S., Sakumoto, D., Itano, K. and Tsubota, T. (1964). Ultrastructure of cercaria of *Clonorchis sinensis*. *Jap. J. Parasit.*, **13**, 339.

Inatomi, S., Tongu, Y., Sakumoto, D., Suguri, S. and Itano, K. (1970a). Ultrastructure of *Schistosoma japonicum*. Recent Advances in Researches on Filariasis and Schistosomiasis in Japan. University of Tokyo Press. 257–289.

Inatomi, S., Tongu, Y., Sakumoto, D., Suguri, S. and Itano, K. (1970b). The ultrastructure of helminth. 4. Cercaria of *Schistosoma japonicum*. *Acta Med. Okayama*, **24**, 205.

Kruidenier, F. J. and Vatter, A. E. (1958). Ultrastructure at the surface of cercariae of *Schistosoma mansoni* and of a Plagiorchioid. (*Tetrapapillatrema coucavocorpa*) *J. Parasit.*, **44**, 42.

Kruidenier, F. J. (1959). Ultrastructure of the excretory system of cercariae. *J. Parasit.*, **45**, 59.

Lautenschlager, E. W. and Cardell, R. R. (1959). Ultrastructure of the surface layers of a strigeid metacercaria, *Diplostomulum trituri* and *on Echinostome* cercaria, *Himasthla quissentensis*. *J. Parasit.*, **45**, (4-2, Supp.). 18.

Lumsden, R. D. and Foor, W. E. (1968). Electron microscopy of *Schistosoma* cercarial muscle. *J. Parasit.*, **54**, 780.

Lyons, K. M. (1969a). Sense organs of monogenean skin parasite ending in a typical cilium. *Parasit.*, **59**, 611.

Lyons, K. M. (1969b). Compound sensilla in monogenean skin parasites. *Parasit.*, **59**, 625.

Morris, G. P. and Threadgold, L. T. (1967). A presumed sensory structure associated with the tegument of *Schistosoma mansoni*. *J. Parasit.*, **53**, 537.

Rees, G. (1967). The histochemistry of the cystogenous gland cells and cyst wall of *Parorchis acanthus* Nicoll, and some details of the morphology and fine structure of the cercaria. *Parasit.*, **57**, 87.

Riessig, M. (1970). Characterization of cell types in the parenchyma of *Schistosoma mansoni*. *Parasit.*, **60**, 273.

Robson, R. T. and Erasmus, D. A. (1970). The ultrastructure, based on steroscan observations, of the oral sucker of the cercaria of *Schistosoma mansoni* with special reference to penetration. *Z. Parasit.*, **35**, 76.

Soparker, M. B. (1921). The cercaria of *Schistosoma spindale*. *Ind. J. Med. Res.*, **9**, 1.

Tongu, Y., Sakumoto, D., Suguri, S., Itano, K., Inatomi, S., and Kamachi, S. (1970). The ultrastructure of helminth. 5. *Cercaria longissima*. *Jap. J. Parasit.*, **19**(2), 128.

Wilson, R. A. (1970). Fine structure of the nervous system and specialized nerve endings in the miracidium of *Fasciola hepatica*. *Parasit.*, **60**, 399.

National Control Program of Filariasis and Schistosomiasis in Japan

T. Ishimaru

Communicable Disease Control Section, Ministry of Health and Welfare of Japan, Tokyo, Japan

INTRODUCTION

Filariasis has long been one of the most important endemic diseases in Japan, causing suffering and disabling effects on large numbers of people living in the southern regions.

Two species of human filariae have been known to be endemic in Japan; *Wuchereria bancrofti* and *Brugia malayi*. The latter was found only on a small island of Hachijo-Koshima, located south of Tokyo. The Malayan filariasis of this type was never found in other areas in Japan during extensive blood surveys carried out in connection with a country-wide filariasis control program.

In the period of disorder that followed World War II, the incidence of ascariasis spread throughout Japan at an increased rate, in the cities as well as farm villages. Another parasitic disease, schistosomiasis japonica, was also on the increase. However, because the size of the area in which filariasis and schistosomiasis were localized, it was not classified and given attention on a national scale and so it was treated more as a local problem for the farming populations in the endemic areas.

Recently, in the last 10 years, positive measures have been taken against filariasis and schistosomiasis japonica, and as a result, both diseases have almost been eradicated in Japan.

The history of the disease control program and its developments in our country up to the present time are outlined in the present paper.

THE NATIONAL FILARIASIS CONTROL PROGRAM

Based on the information and experience accumulated during the past ten years, the government of Japan came to a decision to support a country-wide filariasis control program starting in the fiscal year 1962, and this program was carried out along the guide text for standard methods which was drafted by Sasa and issued by the Ministry of Health and Welfare. The departments of health of local governments were responsible for selecting the areas to be surveyed and treated and for conducting the blood surveys, while the municipalities carried out the drug administration and mosquito control work.

The outline of the methods employed in the filariasis control program in Japan are summarized as follows:

The purpose of this program is to carry out epidemiological surveys for the detection of parasite carriers among the people in endemic areas, and to eradicate the parasite through application of adequate drug treatment schemes. For the prevention of transmission of the disease, it is also intended in the program to undertake the survey and control of vector mosquitoes.

Procedures of filariasis control program

All areas (a) where microfilarial carriers have been demonstrated by previous surveys, (b) where clinical cases have been brought to the attention of physicians, and (c) where occurrence of the disease is suspected, based on other evidence, are suspected as endemic areas.

All people in the areas concerned are to be examined by blood survey, with the exception of infants under 12 months. The people are requested to visit a blood survey station between 9 p.m. and 12 p.m. The 30 cubic mm of blood is drawn into a "filaria pipette" from the earlobe and transferred to a slide in three rows of 10 cubic mm each. The blood smears on the slides are hemolysed by adding tap water and stained with Giemsa solution. In the microscopic examinations of the blood smears, low power magnification should be used, and microfilarial count in each of the 10 cubic mm smears should be recorded for each person. Parasite carriers and clinical cases should be registered.

To all the microfilarial carriers, the drug "diethylcarbabamazine" should be administered. The drug is given once a day, for 12 days, with single doses of 0.3 g in adults, 0.25 g in middle school pupils, and 0.15 g in primary school pupils. As a rule, the total doses given in the course of the treatment are 3.6 g in adults, 3.0 g in middle school pupils and 1.8 g in primary school pupils.

About three months after completion of the initial course of drug treatment, the microfilarial carriers should be reexamined and those who are still positive should receive another course of the drug treatment.

As far as mosquito control methods are concerned, the following items have been adopted: Survey of mosquito fauna and breeding places in the endemic areas concerned. Removal of mosquito breeding places, with emphasis on sewage ditches near houses. Use of mosquito larvicides and natural enemies. Residual spray of insecticides.

THE NATIONAL SCHISTOSOMIASIS CONTROL PROGRAM

Schistosomiasis japonica was known long ago as a strange disease prevalent in limited areas of Hiroshima, Yamanashi and Saga Prefectures. The earliest medical records date back to "Katayama-ki" written by Fujii in 1847. After that, many workers made efforts to clarify the nature of this disease and the life cycle of the parasite. Together with research on preventive measures against the disease, research on the development in the final host, pathogenicity, therapeutics, and such factors, made rapid progress. A more complete picture of the facts and details about the endemic areas in Japan was also drawn up in 1913.

As soon as it became known, in 1913, that *Oncomelania nosophora* acts as the intermediate host, molluscicides such as caustic lime and calcium cyanamide were sprayed throughout endemic areas in an attempt to control the vector snails. Consequently, before World War II the number of snails and the number of cases of schistosomiasis was on the decrease in endemic areas. However, during the war and during the period of disorder following it, implementation of control measures for schistosomiasis was almost impossible; and so in each endemic area the number of cases once again increased rapidly.

In the fiscal year 1950, the local government concerned started the schistosomiasis control program supported financially by the Japanese Government. The methods employed in the schistosomiasis control program are almost the same as those in filariasis control program.

Procedures of the schistosomiasis control program
After information on the host was accumulated, five areas were

mapped out as endemic areas of schistosomiasis japonica:
   the Katayama district in Hiroshima and Okayama Prefectures;
   the Kofu Basin in Yamanashi Prefecture;
   the Chikugo River basin running through Fukuoka and Saga
   Prefectures;
   the Tone River in Chiba, Saitama, and Ibaragi Prefectures;
   the Numazu district in Shizuoka Prefecture.

Among these 5 districts the first 3 districts were adopted in this
control program, as there were no actual patients in the other 2
districts.

All the people willing to take examinations in the areas concerned
were examined for stool by centrifugation method, but before 1965
the direct smear method was used for stool examination.

All egg carriers by stool examination and cases who showed any
clinical symptoms were treated with sodium antimonyl tartalate free
of medical fees.

Since the beginning of this control program, the local government
has required the spraying of sodium pentachlorophenate (NaPCP)
throughout all endemic areas, in an effort to eliminate O. nosophora
as control measure for schistosomiasis and since 1969, instead of

Table 1.   Annual Changes of Notified Cases and Deaths

Year	Schistsomisis japonica		Filariasis	
	Cases	Deaths	Cases	Deaths
1950	918	81	106	59
1951	697	54	71	64
1952	948	71	40	55
1953	1200	73	55	61
1954	1537	86	187	64
1955	1349	80	61	54
1956	1442	74	98	57
1957	664	57	61	53
1958	1983	69	122	46
1959	936	57	39	50
1960	449	41	59	44
1961	430	42	80	38
1962	359	46	1536	31
1963	270	33	126	32
1964	446	31	639	25
1965	228	27	118	33
1966	211	16	14	28
1967	187	21	19	15
1968	95	0	13	0

NaPCP, dibromo-hydroxy-nitroazobenzene (Yurimin) has been used as molluscicide for economy and to spare environmental pollution. The local governments also began lining all irrigation ditches in the rice paddies with concrete.

The annual change of notified cases and deaths in both diseases is presented in Table 1 which is compiled from the statistics of communicable diseases (1969). The surveys under the control program of filariasis and schistosomiasis, such as the examination of the population, detected cases, control activities and expenditures for the programs, are compiled from the official annual reports presented from the Prefectural Governments to the Ministry of Health and Welfare are shown in Tables 2 to 5.

Table 2.   Progress of Filariasis and Schistosomiasis
Control Program in Japan

	Filariasis control			Schistosomiasis control		
Year	Number treated	Number of household insecticide fumigated	Expenditure ¥1,000	Number treated	Area treated with molluscicide (ha)	Expenditure ¥1,000
1962	14,964	187,547	15,795			
1963	8,263	123,328	31,536			
1964	5,540	75,406	20,594	410	4,799	15,442
1965	3,509	64,373	18,119	260	5,088	15,319
1966	2,261	51,691	12,011	309	5,690	14,544
1967	1,490	45,859	7,876	228	5,171	12,821
1968	1,160	39,734	5,044	343	5,064	12,777
1969	4,812	24,477	5,044	239	4,175	10,609

Table 3.   Microfilaria Positive Rate

Year	Population under control	Number examined	Number positive	Percent positive	Expenditure ¥1,000
1962	2,189,114	562,822	15,696	2.8	15,795
1963	2,096,606	507,675	8,278	1.6	31,536
1964	2,270,516	337,891	5,544	1.6	20,594
1965	337,104	167,577	3,517	2.1	18,119
1966	315,763	125,080	2,261	1.8	12,011
1967	283,128	128,331	1,491	1.2	7,876
1968	201,771	93,150	1,160	1.2	5,044
1969	192,125	91,192	441	0.5	5,044

Table 4. Annual Incidence of *Schistosoma japonicum* Infection Based on the Stool Direct Smear Examination

Year	Number examined	Number positive	Percent positive	Expenditure ¥1,000
1963	69,807	191	0.3	6,249
1964	59,268	51	0.1	5,700
1965	49,188	174	0.4	6,457
1966	46,063	124	0.3	5,527
1967	37,206	159	0.4	5,088
1968	45,484	289	0.6	4,952
1969	43,129	161	0.4	4,364

Table 5. The Improvement Plan for Irrigation Ditches in Shistosomiasis Control Project

Local	Total length of irrigation ditches	Length of improved ditches							
		1965	1966	1967	1968	1969	1970	Total	%
Yamanashi	802,488 (m)	150,063	76,724	50,938	62,877	82,416	94,867	517,885	65
Okayama	4,264	720	682	511	584	429	670	3,596	84
Hiroshima	71,505	12,180	9,998	7,942	10,607	5,538	6,310	52,575	74
Fukuoka	197,856	24,394	22,891	17,280	21,647	18,428	23,304	127,944	65
Saga	155,791	21,780	24,030	19,228	9,058	14,381	16,514	104,911	67
Total	1,231,904	209,137	134,325	95,899	104,772	121,112	141,665	806,909	66

REFERENCES

Ministry of Health and Welfare (1969).   Statistics of Communicable Disease and Food Poisoning.

A Historical Review of the Early Japanese Contributions to the Knowledge of Schistosomiasis Japonica*

M. Sasa

*Department of Parasitology, Institute of Medical Science,
University of Tokyo, Tokyo, Japan*

INTRODUCTION

The disease caused by *Schistosoma japonicum* Katsurada (1904) is known to be endemic only in East Asia, i.e. in some parts of Japan, China (including both the mainland and Taiwan), the Philippines, and also in Celebes of Indonesia, Thailand, Laos and Cambodia. Although its geographical distribution is thus restricted, it is a serious health hazard to a large number of people residing in the endemic areas, as was pointed out by Faust and Meleney (1924), Stoll (1947), Wright (1950) and a number of other workers. At least 5% of the world's population are estimated to reside in the endemic areas often associated with high infection rates. The infection frequently causes serious symptoms by involvement of digestive tract, liver and even the brain. Of the three major schistosome species causing disease in man, *S. japonicum* is considered to be the most severe pathogen, and is unusual among the helminths in that it frequently kills the host.

While schistosomiasis japonica is now known to be distributed over a vast range extending several thousands of kilometers, the most essential facts pertaining to this disease were worked out through the painstaking efforts of early Japanese medical scientists and physicians during the twenty years' period from near the end of last century to about 1915. These include the establishment as a previously unknown disease, discovery of the causative agent, the mode of infection of man

---

* This study was conducted while a Fogarty Scholar-in-Residence, Fogarty International Center, NIH. Thanks are due to Dr. Paul P. Weinstein, the University of Notre Dame, to Dr. James F. Haggerty and Mrs. Marion Leech of Fogarty International Center, NIH, for valuable advice and assistance, and to Dr. G. Burroughs Mider and staff of the National Library of Medicine for providing facilities in conducting this study.

and animals, and the entire life history in the intermediate and final hosts. However, these historically important contributions were published mostly in Japanese and in periodicals generally inaccessible to workers other than in Japan. Even Japanese scientists of my age or younger know little about this history. While I was working on a review of this and other diseases endemic in Asia at the National Library of Medicine, Bethesda, I thought it would be worthwhile to review these early contributions which had been only poorly publicized by previous workers. Fortunately, this library has almost complete collections of the classical western medical papers, many of which were inaccessible to me while I was in Japan, and at the same time a fairly good collection of even the old Japanese periodicals pertaining to this field of research.

A map of the endemic areas af schistosomiasis in Japan is attached to the last page.

1. *Recognition of the Disease: the earliest stage.*

Schistosomiasis japonica is a disease recognized rather recently in the history of medicine. While there are records of the recognition of schistosomiasis haematobia during the reign of Pharaoh in Egypt, and its presence in mummies (1250 to 100 B.C.) has been confirmed, exact knowledge regarding schistosomiasis japonica evolved rather recently. The earliest record dealing with this desease is considered to be *Katayama-ki* by YOSHINAO FUJII in 1847.

Katayama-ki is a record prepared by a physician residing near an endemic area of this disease in western Honshu, Japan. It was written with a brush and Chinese ink on indigenous Japanese paper (washi) in a classical Chinese grammar (kanbun), when the author was 33 years old. Fujii was born at Yamate-son, which is now a part of Fukuyama City, Hiroshima Prefecture, where he spent most of his life as a practicing physician. It was the era of Tokugawa, or before Japan underwent her cultural revolution of Meiji, and the rulers at that time strictly prohibited the introduction of western medicine. Although many authors cite that *Katayama-ki* was published in 1847 in a journal (Chugai Iji Shimpo, No. 691, pp. 55–56), this is not true. It was written in 1847, but was published by Professor Fujinami in this journal in 1909, with his comments. The original copy had been kept at Fujinami's laboratory in Kyoto University, but was unfortunately lost by fire.

Since *Katayama-ki* is considered important not only as the oldest medical record referring to schistosomiasis japonica, but also has stimulated many workers with the need for research on this desease, it is intended here to present an almost full translation. The original was written in *kanbun* (classical Chinese grammar), which was the official way of writing a document at that time, and thus some parts are difficult to understand even for me.

"There is a village called Kawanami in the south of Kannabe-eki of western Bingo county. There are two hills called Ikariyama and Katayama, which are surrounded by rice paddies. The latter is known also as Urushi-yama. It is said that in olden times while this area was a bay, a boat loaded with urushi* trees was wrecked by a strong wind on the shore of this hill. Thereafter, people who passed nearby this hill acquired *urushi*-dermatitis. Actually, I have seen during the pa t couple of years, people suffering from severe itches associated with small rashes on the legs. All were those who had entered water of these rice paddies. The same happened to horses and cattle. The people here are convinced that the disease is caused by the poison of *urushi*. There are also many patients showing such signs as diarrhea, jaundice, emaciation, and rapid pulse. There are also cases of debility, severe diarrhea, tenesmus and bloody stool. In the advanced stage, the legs and hands become extremely thin, while only the belly is swollen like a drum. The veins on the breasts are highly dilated, the navel protrudes, and sometimes the abdominal wall become so thin and transparent that the intestine is seen through it. Finally, they get oedema of the legs, and die. I do not know what disease this is. It looks like "consumption" initially, but develops into "enlargement of abdomen" at the last stage. The patients are various ages, from 7 or 8 years to 40 or 50 years. There are also mild cases, which are not confined to bed and recover within a few months to a year. In severe cases, even strong men acquire the disease and die. They use various medicines, but none of them are effective. I have already seen over 30 deaths. Some 50 cattle and horses have also died. The area around Katayama is most severe, but people also contract the disease in areas near Ikariyama. The disease occurs in two other valleys in this area, and also in the neighboring villages of Senda. I cannot clarify the cause of this disease by any means. Is it really due to the poison of *urushi* or caused by some agent in the rice paddy water? Although Katayama is several miles distant from the sea, the early literature indicates that this area was once a bay and that the mast of a wrecked boat was found while digging a well. Whether the disease is connected with these events is not certain"

June 1847, by Yoshinao Fujii

There is another record written by Fujii 30 years later under the title of "*Katayama-saiki*", in which he states:

"While I was reviewing old papers, I found my previous manuscript of *Katayama-ki*. Thirty years have passed since then. Although the disease has become less prevalent, there are still some people dying. The people working in the rice paddy

---

Urushi is a Japanese name for Oriental lacquer, made from the *urushi*-tree, *Rhus vernicifera*. The lacquer as well as the tree itself contains a poison that causes severe dermatitis, called *urushi-kabure* (lacquer dermatitis).

still suffer from the itch during the spring-summer season. There is a hard tumor palpable below the breast in all those who have experienced the dermatitis, irrespective of their age. People call it "Katayama disease." Although its symptoms vary greatly among the patients, its causative agent must be the small bugs that give rise to the rash on the legs. This is really a horrible agent. Medical science has made great progress over the years, and new tools have become available. It is told that the western medicine has developed some analytical methods. I hope the analysis of the soil will be carried out with these techniques to find out what kind of poison in the water would cause the disease. Otherwise, there is no way to prevent the disease. I am writing this again to call for assistance of every scholar for solution of this problem."——

Unfortunately, no solution to the problem was given before Fujii died in 1895. However, as Professor Fujinami stated while citing *Katayama-ki* in the medical journal in 1909, Fujii's description of the disease and the assumption of its cause were quite accurate and correct, and have stimulated the interest of many later workers to engage in researches on this disease. The causative agent was discovered nearly 10 years after Fujii's death, and it took 10 additional years before "the small bug in the rice paddy water" was identified as the cercaria of *Schistosoma japonicum*. The eradication of schistosomiasis from Katayama area was achieved in about 1955, as the first among the endemic areas in Japan and elsewhere in the world, by efforts of a number of workers who followed through with Fujii's idea.

Sporadic reports or records are available from other endemic areas in Japan referring to this disease before it was established as a parasitic infection. People in Yamanashi called the disease *suishu-choman*, which means oedema and big belly, and recognized it as *chiho-byo* (endemic, or localized disease) peculiar to this district. Dr. Saburo Sugiura of Yamanashi has told me about a number of tragic stories or folk songs handed down from old time, such as "*suishu choman chawan no kakera*" (there are no means of recovering from the disease, as with the broken cup), or such songs as "A bride marrying the farmer of endemic area must carry a coffin along." There is a written document submitted by a village chief of the endemic area to the governor of Yamanashi Prefecture in 1881. "In Komatsu of Kasugai-mura, several villagers pass away every year suffering from *suishu-choman*. Even the physicians do not know what the cause is, and no drug has ever been effective against this disease. Since all the villagers are very much worried about it, I am requesting that official action be taken by the Govenor to investigate this disease which is endemic in our area."

In our present knowledge, the disease in Japan is endemic in roughly five zones completely isolated from each other, but from the earliest stage of the investigation until about 1904, the disease had been studied independently at each locality, especially in the Katayama area of Hiroshima, in the Kofu area of Yamanashi, and in the Chikugo River basin of Saga-Fukuoka Prefectures. The need for research on this desease was officially recognized in the Katayama area as early as 1882, and a "committee on Katayama disease" was organized. However, results of the investigations carried out by medical workers in this and other areas considered that this was the liver fluke or a malaria-like disease (Nakahama 1884, Oka 1886), or the hookworm disease (Nagamachi, 1887). In the meantime, Majima (1888) reported on the autopsy of a patient who died in a hospital in Tokyo, under the title "A curious liver cirrhosis due to parasite eggs." (The handwritten figures of the liver histology as well as the eggs are now considered typical of schistosomiasis, but no previous history of the patient's residence nor his relation to the endemic area was mentioned). In a discussion, the author states that the findings were most closely related to those reported for *Distomum haematobium* in Africa. The parasite's name was left undetermined.

YAMAGIWA (1889, 1890, 1891) in Tokyo gave detailed accounts of the pathological findings at autopsy in the brain or liver of Jackson's epilepsy and liver cirrhosis caused by the embolism of "a distoma egg," but he thought it was due to the lung fluke. (These cases were confirmed later by Yamagiwa, 1909, as schistosomiasis.)

Meanwhile, the idea that the disease in these endemic areas might be due to a new parasite gradually evolved. KURIMOTO (1893), while visiting Saga Prefecture in Kyushu for a survey of the liver fluke disease, found "a new parasite egg" in the liver of two patients who died of liver cirrhosis, and pointed out that in addition to the already known liver fluke disease, there was another new parasitic disease in this area. Five years later, KANAMORI (1898) reported on a female patient with advanced liver cirrhosis hospitalized in Tokyo. She was a resident of Yamashiro-mura, Yamanashi; at autopsy numerous eggs of "a new parasite" was discovered in the liver. He recognized various differential characters between this and the eggs of the lung fluke, especially the absence of operculum in the former. Upon re-examination of the preserved specimens, he confirmed that some of the cases reported as having lung fluke eggs in the tissues by Yamagiwa (1889, 1890), Matsushima (1895) and Suzuki (1895), as well as those with unknown or new prasite eggs described by Majima (1888) and Kurimoto (1893) were the same parasitic disease. He further found four cases of liver cirrhosis due to this parasite egg among specimens preserved at the Pathology Department of the University of Tokyo. It is stated in this article that "I asked identification of this egg to Professor Iijima at the Department of Zoology. He said that this would probably be a nematode egg. He further pointed out that he had seen the same eggs in Kurimoto's specimen."

Kanamori was probably the first who associated the endemic disease of Yamanashi with this "new parasite egg." This important finding aroused profound concern in medical workers in Yamanashi (MURAKAMI, 1902; MUKOYAMA, 1902). NIIZUMA (1902, 1903) at the Yamanashi Prefectural Hospital confirmed the presence of "Kanamori's new eggs" in the liver and intestine of three autopsy cases each having typical symptoms of the endemic disease. In the meantime, MIKAMI (1900, 1901, 1904), MIURA (1904, 1905) and TSUCHIYA (1904–1906) in Yamanashi collected extensive information on the epidemiological and clinical aspects of this desease. KURIMOTO (1904) also pointed out the presence in Yamanashi of the same disease he had found in Saga in 1893.

On the other hand, Kasai (1904) discovered eggs of an unfamiliar parasite in feces of a patient from Katayama area admitted to Kyoto University Hospital. He thought this might be the cause of Katayama disease, and carried out an extensive survey of this area. Case reports were made on 29 patients with advanced symptoms. He also conducted physical examination of the general population, and found swelling of the liver or spleen in 44 of 193 people in Katayama Village and in 22 of 56 people in Oji Village. At stool examinations, he found the same unfamiliar eggs in 2 of 7 cases. After taking various factors into consideration, he assumed that the parasite would possibly be the cause of Katayama disease. (According to his figures, the eggs are definitely those of *S. japonicum*). He observed the hatching of a larva under the microscope when warm water was added. The size of these eggs according to his measurement was 0.109–0.081 mm in length and 0.0765–0.0533 in width, and thus it was significantly larger than those reported by Kanamori (1898) from the tumor (0.0810–0.0624 in length, 0.0546–0.0312 in width) or in the liver (0.0720–0.0540 in length, 0.0540–0.0360 in width). The content of the eggs was also quite different; the former in stool had a larva, while the latter was described as evenly granular. Therefore, Kasai could not associate his eggs in the stool with those in the tissues reported by Kanamori and others. (In our present concept, those in tissues are mostly degenerated eggs, and also eggs become larger when discharged with the stool, but Kasai's measurement is still too large).

Autopsies and histological examinations of Katayama disease were finally carried out by Maki and Maruyama (1904) and by Fujinami and Kon (1904). Through detailed studies of these materials, Fujinami (1904) confirmed that the disease endemic in Katayama and Yamanashi was caused by the same parasite.

2. Discovery of the parasite

After going through such a long course of investigations on the cause of this disease, and while most of the leading workers at that time became convinced that the disease was caused by an unknown parasite, Katsurada (1904 a, b), who was the professor of pathology at Okayama Medical College, finally discovered the adult worm and determined the disease as a new schistosomiasis. He became interested in this disease through the results reported by other workers, and visited Yamanashi for a period from April 6 to 10, 1904. Assisted by Mikami and a number of other local physicians, he made a survey of the endemic area, and examined 12 cases with typical signs of the endemic disease. From stool examinations of these patients, he found a peculiar type of egg in 4 cases, and identified it as belonging to the blood fluke group, based on such characters as the presence of a miracidium and the lack of an operculum on the egg shell. He also made an assumption that the adult worms must be residing not in the intestinal canal but probably in the intestinal wall or other organs connected with it, because the eggs were not always found in the patients and become more abundant after administration of a purgative. He further examined material from three autopsies preserved at the local hospital, and confirmed the presence of the same eggs in the liver and other organs.

While visiting the endemic area, Katsurada was interested in examining some animals, since he had known from his past experience with liver and lung flukes that the parasites could be found also in cats and dogs. He sacrificed a cat and three dogs, brought the autopsied materials to the laboratory in Okayama, and recovered a single male worm from the portal vein of the cat; the dogs were negative. This was identified as an undescribed species of schistosome. These results were published in two journals, in Okayama Igakkai Zasshi on 30 June, and in Tokyo Iji Shinshi in two series, on August 6 and 13, 1904.

Encouraged by these results, Katsurada made a second visit to Yamanashi on July 25 of the same year. He obtained one cat already showing advanced signs of the disease. In the liver, there were numerous eggs of the same kind as were found in the human cases. From the portal vessels, he recovered 24 male and 8 female worms. These were closely related to the already known human blood fluke, *S. haematobium* (Bilharz, 1852), but he found several characters definitely separating the species. The manuscript referring to this study was mailed to Tokyo Iji Shinshi on August 6, and appeared as an addendum to his report on August 13. As a conclusion to this article, Katsurada stated "I want to use, for the time being, the name *Schistosomum japonicum* for this parasite." So long as he gave the latin binomial names, morphological description and a differential diagnosis, this article should be recognized as the original description of this species, though Katsurada (1904 g) later published a more comprehensive description of this parasite with designation as a new species.

In the meantime, Catto (1905) while staying in a quarantine station in Singapore, conducted an autopsy of a Chinese man who came from Fukien and had died of cholera on a boat, and found numerous eggs in liver and other organs. After returning to England, he further examined the material, found both male and female worms in blood vessels, and named it *Schistosoma cattoi*. This was published in the British Medical Journal on January 7, 1905, about 5 months later than Katsurada's *S. japonicum* though dealing with the same species.

The discovery of the adult worm in man was achieved by Fujinami (1904) at his second autopsy carried out on May 30, 1904. The patient was a 53 year old male, who was murdered in Katayama and was subjected to forensic autopsy. Fujinami brought the material to his laboratory, and after a long and painstaking search of various organs, finally obtained a single female worm from a branch of the portal vein in the left lobe of the liver. The eggs identical with those found free in the patient's organs were seen in its uterus. He identified this worm as to be closely related to *Bilharzia haematobia*. The paper was read at a meeting held on September 17, and was published in the October 15 issue of Tokyo Iji Shinshi. Fujinami later confirmed that the parasite in man and those described from cats by Katsurada (1904 b) as *S. japonicum* were the same, and thus the cause of the

endemic disease of Katayama and Yamanashi areas was unequivo-
cally established. Additional recoveries of numerous adult worms
from human cases were reported by Tsuchiya (1906) from Yamanashi, and by Fujinami (1907) and Nakamura (1910) from Katayama districts. In animals, Tsuchiya found the adults in cats (1904)
and also in dogs (1905), and Nozaki (1905), Fujinami (1907) and
Nakamura (1910) found the infection in calves of Katayama.

Another important contribution achieved by Katsurada (1904 a)
at that time was the establishment of a diagnostic method by examination of schistosome eggs in the stool. Katsurada (1904 c) made a
survey of the Saga area in August 1904, found schistosome eggs in
stools of 2 of 3 patients he examined, and confirmed that the so-called
"curious endemic disease" in Saga was also schistosomiasis japonica.
(In the present reviewer's view, Katsurada far exceeded other workers at that time in the knowledge and experience in parasitology,
though the others might have been more expert in pathology or
clinical medicine. As stated above, he was the first who diagnosed
the eggs to be characteristic of a blood fluke based on the absence of
an operculum and by its content being a miracidium. He further
predicted the infection in animals and the presence of adult worms in
the portal vein.)

Note: Recognition of schistosomiasis japonica in other countries.

Following the reports by Katsurada (1904) from Japan and by
Catto (1905) from Singapore, in a Chinese from Fukien, the occurrence of schistosomiasis japonica in some other Oriental countries
became established. Those who first reported the disease in their respective countries were Logan (1905) from mainland China, Wooley
(1906) from the Philippines, Takegami (1914) from Taiwan, Brug
& Tesch (1937) from Celebes, Galliard (1957) from Laos, Chaiyaporn
(1959) from southern Thailand, and Audebaud *et al.* (1968) from
Cambodia.

3. *The mode of infection*

The next question which remained unresolved was the mode of
infection, and the developmental cycle of the parasite. There were
differences of opinion among the workers at that time, as to whether
the parasite would infect man by way of mouth or through the skin,
and whether or not it would require an intermediate host. The life
cycle of *Schistosoma haematobium* in Egypt was still unknown and various hypotheses had been raised also by European scholars at this

stage of research. As for the route of invasion of the parasite, most workers seemed to be more in favor of the oral rather than the cutaneous route, because theoretically the former offered a better explanation of the presence of adult worms in the intestinal and protal vessels. However, epidemiological evidence and experience of the farmers in the endemic areas suggested the possibility of cutaneous infection, as was described by Fujii in his *Katayama-saiki*.

For instance, Katsurada (1904 a) in a discussion stated that "not only the drinking of water contaminated with the parasite, but also exposure of the skin in the rice paddy water might be dangerous." He furhter pointed out that there were two different kinds of dermatitis occurring among the farmers in Yamanashi; one was called *mizu-kabure* (water dermatitis), which appeared on the middle part of the legs corresponding to the site of contact with the water surface while the farmers were working in the rice paddies. The other was called *koe-kabure* (night soil dermatitis), which occurred chiefly between the toes after the farmers spent some time in the vegetable fields where night soil had been applied thickly. (This was an important epidemiological finding recognized by Katsurada. In our present concept, the former is caused by invasion of schistosome cercariae, and the latter by hookworm larvae.)

Tsuchiya (1904 a), on the other hand, strongly opposed Katsurada's view. "I am convinced that there is no relationship between the dermatitis and the endemic disease. The dermatitis must be caused by some chemical substances produced by decomposition of the night soil. If the parasite invades through the skin, the adult worms must be found in all vessels. In the cats I examined, there were no worms in vessels other than the portal system."

In this study, Tsuchiya observed that when feces obtained from infected man or cats were preserved in water, the eggs hatched and the larvae began to swim actively in water. Since the larvae soon died in physiological saline, he presumed that they would infect man by way of the mouth after passing through a development either in an intermediate host, or by growing in water. Tsuchiya and Toyama (1905) again emphasized the need for improvement of water supply and sterilization of food as the major preventive measures.

In the meantime, Fujinami (1907) carried on pathological studies in the Katayama area, and reported on the recovery of 4 male and 5 female worms from his third autopsy case from Katayama, as well as on the pathological findings in infected cats, dogs and cattle. On the basis of the site of recovery of the adult worms, he assumed the route of infection was probably by way of the mouth, but added that the possibility of invasion through the skin must not be entirely rejected. Prior to this, Katsurada (1906) also stated that, "Although certain numbers of the larvae might invade through the skin, this would probably be an unusual route of infection; it is assumed that the majority of them reach the mesenteric vessels by way of the digestive canal, especially through the wall of the small intestine."

In order to test their hypotheses, the workers of both groups carried out field experiments in 1909, rather independently but with similar methods. The results reported by Katsurada and Hasegawa (1909) as well as by Fujinami and Nakamura (1909) agreed in that the infection could take place through the skin, by exposure of animals to the water where people frequently contracted the dermatitis. The former group of workers visited a newly discovered endemic area in Okayama Prefecture (Tagami Village of Oeson) on June 11, 1909, and immersed one cat in a ditch, and a dog in a rice paddy water, both for about 3 hours once a day for three consecutive days, June 12 to 15. The animals were brought from non-endemic areas, fed only with sterilized food and water, and their head was fixed with a large plate during exposure to the water so that they were not allowed to drink the contaminated water. Both animals were brought back to their laboratory in Okayama Medical College. The cat became positive for schistosome eggs at the beginning of July, about one month after the exposure, and died on July 26. On autopsy, numerous adult worms were found in the portal vessels. The dog also became ill at the beginning of July, began to pass numerous eggs in the stool, but was still alive at the time they submitted the paper (this article appeared in the August 31, 1909, issue of Okayama Igakkai Zasshi).

The experiments conducted by Fujinami and Nakamura (1909) in Katayama were more comprehensive and larger in scale. A committee for the study of endemic disease in Katayama was organized, and a group of workers visited the area from Kyoto on June 1, two weeks earlier than Katsurada and Hasegawa initiated their experiment. (Since Fujinami and associates had to pass through Okayama on their travel from Kyoto to Katayama, it is probable that Fujinami's idea had been communicated to Katsurada.) In their main experiment, they used 17 calves brought from a non-endemic area, and to determine whether the parasite invades orally or cutaneously, the animals were divided into the following four groups:

Group A: Composed of 6 calves, of which 3 were exposed to water
of Takase River (Group A-1), while the other 3 (Group A-2) were
taken to irrigation ditches and rice paddies, daily for several hours a
day for about 40 days from about June 10. The mouth of each animal
of these groups was covered with a special bag so that the animal
could not drink the polluted water nor eat the grass in the fields, and
all their food and drinking water were provided after being sterilized
by heat. The legs only were exposed to the polluted waters.

Group B: 7 calves were used, of which 3 (Group B-1) were brought
to the bank of the river every day the same as group A-1, and the
other 4 (Group B-2) were brought to the same site as the group A-2;
they were allowed to graze or to drink the presumably polluted grass
or water freely, but their legs were covered with special water-proof
boots so that their skin would never be exposed to the water. Whenever any part of their body came in contact with the water, this was
washed and the body part was sterilized with alcohol.

Group C: 2 calves, fed with the sterilized food and water the same
as for the group A, and kept all through the experimental period in a
cow shed.

Group D: 2 calves, brought to the river bank every day, the same
as for Group A-1 and B-1. They were allowed to graze or drink water,
and also to expose the skin to the polluted waters.

Nine calves among them were sacrificed and autopsied during the
period from July 3 to 20 while they were in Katayama, and the other
8 calves were shipped to their laboratory in Kyoto on July 26 for
further observations. The results were quite conclusive. All the animals of Groups A and D whose legs were exposed to the water were
heavily infected. In group A-2 exposed to the ditches and rice paddies, the worm burden was the highest, and several thousand adults
were recovered, whereas those exposed to the river water were much
lower in infection. In the animals of Groups B and C whose legs were
protected from exposure to the polluted waters, no infection was
observed, with the exception of one animal which harbored only one
parasite. Grazing or drinking of the possibly polluted materials did
not cause the infection. They also succeeded in infecting 9 dogs and
one rabbit by exposure to ditches or rice paddies in the endemic
area, and obtained various developmental stages of the parasite from
the portal vein.

These experiments carried out by Fujinami and Nakamura are
historically important not only in that they demonstrated unequiv-

ocally the route of infection of this parasite, but also in the sense that subsequently animal experiments with this parasite became feasible for other workers. By this report, it was shown for the first time that laboratory animals like the rabbit were also susceptible.

Although it was demonstrated here that the parasite could invade the skin while exposed to the infested water, nobody at that time had seen the infective form of the schistosome, and it was also questionable whether the water dermatitis (*kabure*) was due to the invasion of the larva. Umeda (1909) presented a series of papers in which he claimed that *kabure* was possibly caused by a kind of Ciliata (probably *Paramecium*) which he found abundantly in the infested waters, and bore no relation to schistosomiasis nor to chemical substances from night soil. (although his assumption was incorrect, he gave valuable information on the occurrence of *kabure* in relation to the environment based on his observations in Katayama.)

Another important contribution was made by Matsuura (1909) of the Dermatology Department of Kyoto University, who confirmed the route of infection in man by his own experience. Like most other workers at that time, he was also very suspicious about the relationship between the dermatitis and contraction of the disease such as claimed by people in the endemic areas. He visited Katayama area for the first time from June 27 to July 1, 1908. At that time, he and some other volunteers entered rice paddies and ditches several times to experience *kabure* themselves, but the results were negative, i.e. nobody exhibited such a reaction. The second visit was during August 11 to 18 of the same year, and again no *kabure* occurred. He stated that this might have been due to heavy rain which washed away the causative agents. In the next year, he made the third visit during June 15 to 27. After several unsuccessful trials, he finally contracted *kabure* on June 20, while he was standing in a rice paddy at Nakatsuhara. However, this occurred only on his bare left leg. The other leg, on which he exhibited no reaction, was covered with a thick cloth (gaiter). On June 22, he again exposed both legs in the water, covering one leg with a cotton cloth (*tenjuku-momen*) and the other with a mosquito net cloth. *Kabure* occurred only on the latter. On June 24, he again exposed the legs after smearing lard on one leg and camellia oil on the other. There was no reaction on both of his legs, while *kabure* occurred on all other volunteers who received no such treatments. There were many discussions about the nature of *kabure* among the co-workers. Some thought that it was merely due to the bite of water leeches, whereas others were in favor of some chemical poisons. But Matsuura demonstrated that the causative agent was not a chemical poison nor a big animal, but was something which could penetrate through the mesh of mosquito net but not through cotton cloth, and could be repelled by a barrier of lard or some oil.

There is another important story about Matsuura's experiment. After he came back to Kyoto, he began to feel weak from about the middle of July, but he thought this was due to the hot climate. However, the sick feeling became worse, and he did not recover until the end of August, even when the climate became cooler. Then he was suddenly reminded of his past experience. On examination of his stool on September 1, three schistosome eggs were found. Later, he gradually recovered from the sick feeling, but he remained positive for eggs for some time thereafter.

(It is presumed that, like most other workers, Matsuura could hardly believe that the parasite, being a trematode, would infect man through the skin. In this article, he states that he strictly boiled all the food and drinking water while staying in Katayama, so as to avoid infection that might take place through the mouth. As a dermatologist, he was probably more interested in clarifying the nature of *kabure*, rather than to associate it with Katayama disease. That is why he did not realize he had contracted the disease until he examined his stool some time after he became ill.)

Fujinami and associates conducted investigations on this desease from various aspects. Yagi (1909–10) reported on the presence of a hemolytic substance in the ether extract of the adult worms. Yoshimoto (1909–10) carried out a complement fixation test of sera from infected and non-infected individuals with an alcoholic extract of the adult worms as the antigen, and obtained satisfactory results as the means of diagnosis. Fujinami and Nakamura (1909) obtained satisfactory results as the means of diagnosis. Fujinami and Nakamura (1909) obtained similar results in the complement fixation test of the calves infected with *Schistosoma*. By 1911, Fujinami and associates found that not only rabbits, but also monkeys, guinea pigs and white rats were susceptible to the infection.

By 1913, Tsuchiya also was obliged to acknowledge the cutaneous route of infection as a result of his own experiments. In an introduction, he mentioned that although people in the Katayama area might have been convinced from old times that the disease agent would invade through the skin, nobody in Yamanashi area had believed it (including himself), and took it for granted that their endemic desease was caused by drinking the polluted water. Therefore, he carried out a public experiment. He shipped large numbers of dogs from Tokyo, which were then kept in a yard of a school in Kofu City. They were divided into two groups. Group A was fed with the water brought every day from irrigation ditches, and the group B animals were immersed into the same water for various periods. All 32 dogs of group B were found to be infected, while none were infected of the 30 dogs fed with the polluted water, even though some had received as much as over 30 liters of the water (Tsuchiya, 1913).

4. *The mode of development in the final host.*

After Fujinami and others had demonstrated that the parasite infects animals in water through the skin, two phases of the life cycle still remained to be clarified: the phase in water from hatching of the miracidium to animal infection, and how the parasite would reach the portal vein system after invasion through the skin. The latter phase of the parasite's development was elucidated by Miyagawa (1912) earlier than the phase in water. He stayed in a village in Yamanashi from May to October 1911, and selected a stream in Nakakomagori (Ikedamura) as the experimental area, since people in this village had been known to be heavily infected. He immersed dogs and rabbits into the stream for 3 to 6 hours daily, for 3 to 8 days. Then, from 2 to 24 hours after the exposure, he took blood from the *vena femoralis* or *vena saphena*, and examined it by two methods; 1) Thick blood smears were allowed to dry on a slide, fixed by flame, and washed in distilled water. The slide was stained with borax carmine, methylene blue, or hematoxylin-eosin. He found worms on a number of slides. 2) 5 to 10 ml of the venous blood was mixed with 50–60 ml of saline in a Petri dish, and after about 2 hours the sediment was examined. He found numerous young worms in good physiological condition.

With the same methods, he recovered various stages of the more developed parasite from the heart blood and the portal vein blood. Examination of some 20,000 histological sections enabled him to demonstrate a few of the earliest stages of the parasite which had just penetrated the skin. Morphological descriptions of the young forms was presented in detail (Faust, 1924, pointed out some of his mistakes). The youngest form found in the skin and in the peripheral venous blood was about 0.04 mm long and 0.015–0.022 mm wide, and possessed various primitive organs, including oral and vental suckers, digestive canal, etc. He further pointed out that there was a difference in size and structure between the young worm just after invasion and the miracidium obtained from the egg. In his measurements, the latter was about 0.1 mm long and 0.04 mm wide, or about 4 times larger than the former. From these observations, Miyagawa concluded that miricidia hatched from eggs did not invade the final host directly, but required some intermediate host to become infective. Through these and later experiments, he confirmed that the parasite, after invading the skin, reached the blood stream either directly, or via the lymphatic system, and finally established itself in the portal system after circulating in the blood stream.

Later, there were some discussions among Japanese scholars on the course of migration of the parasite in the final host. It had been agreed until then, that the young forms after invading the skin, reached the peripheral veins either directly or via the lymphatic system, and later arrive at the right chamber of the heart, as was shown by Miyagawa (1912–13). After the young worms reached the lung, Narabayashi (1916) and Sueyasu (1920) observed that many of the parasites penetrated the lung and appeared in the pleural cavity; thus, they considered that the worms reached the liver or the mesenteric vein from outside, i.e. penetrating through the diaphragm. However, Miyagawa and Takemoto (1921) carried out further detailed experiments in mice, and claimed that these worms were the aberrant ones and that normally they go through the lung capillaries, return to the left heart, and are carried through the aorta to the wall of gastrointestinal tract. Subsequently, they reach their permanent location in the portal vein.

The occurrence of congenital infection in schistosomiasis, confirmed and worked out in detail by Narabayashi (1914–16), is another important aspect of the behavior of the parasite after invasion of the final host. Dogs, rabbits, white rats, guinea pigs and mice were used in his experiments. The pregnant animals were exposed to the infection by immersion into the infested water, and were autopsied at various intervals. Abortion occurred frequently in these animals. He found infection of the parasite in some embryos or new born animals, and the numbers of the worms recovered from the offspring varied from 0.1% to 10% of those found in the mothers. Young schistosomes were found in the histological sections of some of the placenta of guinea pigs. Narabayashi carried out in the Katayama area fecal examinations of 22 babies whose mothers had been estimated to be exposed to infection during pregnancy, and found 3 positives using an egg concentration technique.

Meanwhile, Miyagawa (1912 b) while examining the reaction of host animals at the site of the invasion of larvae, raised serious questions about the relation between *kabure* and the infection with the parasite, since he could not find dermatitis in the animals as was seen in the farmers of the endemic areas. However, Narabayashi (1916) carried out extensive epidemiological surveys and animal experiments to elucidate the relationship and concluded that *kabure* was a reaction specific to the invasion of the parasite, though he also admitted that some animals and man became infected without exhibiting such a reaction. [Schistosome dermatitis is now considered a hypersensitivity reaction in man or animal sensitized by repeated infections; thus both observations are considered acceptable. The reason that Matsuura (1909) did not experience *kabure* in the first year and it appeared in the second year might be due to the fact that he was sensitized by the first year's exposure.]

5. *Discovery of the intermediate host.*

Despite tremendous effort by a number of workers at that time, it still remained unsolved whether or not the parasite utilized an intermediate host for its larval development, and in what form the infective agents occurred in water. As discussed before, most workers predicted the presence of some intermediate host, but none of the investigators could identify it. Fujinami (1916) stated in his review that he invited Mr. Koizumi, a zoologist graduated from the University of Tokyo, to look for all the possible animals in Katayama area, but his efforts were in vain. Both Miyagawa (1913 a) and Tsuchiya (1913 a) stated later that they suspected *kawanina* (*Melania*) to be the most probable intermediate host. By that time, Matsuura & Yamamoto (1911 a, b) by histological study succeeded in demonstrating the worms that had just invaded the skin, and further obtained "the same worm" from the water of a ditch in Katayama area. They immersed animals in a ditch, and collected water with a pipette from near the body of the animal. The water was filtered on a fine mesh cloth (kanakin), and the cloth was washed in 10% formalin, which was then centrifuged. They could not find the worm by direct microscopic examination, but found a few worms in histological sections. [A drawing in their article (Fig. 6) seems to show the body and a part of the tail of a cercaria.]

In the meantime, discovery of the intermediate host was achieved by Miyairi and Suzuki (1913) of Kyushu University, who had just initiated their research in a separate endemic area of northern Kyushu, and a complete understanding of the mode of larval development was reached by their succeeding studies (Miyairi, 1913, 1914; Miyairi and Suziki, 1914). Their first report appeared in Japanese in a weekly journal Tokyo Iji-shinshi, No. 1836, dated September 13, 1913, and Miyairi gave additional comments in No. 1839 of the same journal issued on October 4. In these two papers, they presented some detailed accounts of how the intermediate host was discovered, and how they were delighted by this discovery.

> "We became interested in this subject just several months ago, from the beginning of this year. First of all, we wanted to see the endemic sites, and whenever we had time, we used to walk around the areas in Mitsui-gun, Fukuoka Prefecture. While walking through the villages, we picked up human and animal feces to see the prevalence of schistosomiasis. We also wanted to carry out some animal experiments such as other workers were doing, and looked for adequate places where it might be highly infective. In the meantime, we were taught by a farmer that one of the ditches in that village was famous among the inhabitants to be causing the dermatitis. Then, we went there, and put cats and rabbits into the water, hoping that they would become infected. While we were waiting, we recognized by accident, the presence of a number of snails in the ditch. We brought them to the laboratory, and found out that they could be kept alive for many days in water by providing cabbage as their food.
>
> One day, we tried to see what happens when we put miricidia and the snail together. To our surprize, while swimming in the water, the miracidia became suddenly excited when a snail was introduced, and chased the snail circling around it for a while. Then, once the miricidia attached to the soft part of a snail, either an antenna, head, leg or mantle, they tried to push into the body, and finally all succeeded in penetrating into it. This scene was just the same as that described by Leuckart on the phenomenon he saw with the miracidia of *Fasciola hepatica* and its intermediate host, *Limnaeus minutus*.
>
> We further examined the infected snails. In a lot infected on July 20, we found "the first redia" in their body after 12 days, together with various growth stages of sporocysts. After several weeks, we found that some of the rediae were haboring "second generation rediae," and again these contained "type A" cercariae. [this statement was obviously misled by the finding of Leuckart in *Fasciola hepatica*, in which the larva passes four developmental stages, sporocyst, 1st redia, 2nd redia and cercaria; in the second paper by Miyairi (1913 b), he stated that there was no second redia, but still what they considered a redia at that time was the daughter sporocyst]
>
> On the other hand, we have also observed that most of the adult snails collected in nature harbored cercariae. There are three kinds of cercariae, which we would like to identify tentatively as types A, B, and C. Among them, type A is the most common cercariae. One day, just by chance and without expecting further results, we put a mouse in water containing type A cercariae, for 3 hours. We repeated it for 4 days. In

the morning of August 11, about 3 weeks after the exposure, we found that the mouse was killed by another mouse. Upon dissection, we were very surprised by the unexpected discovery of a large number of adult worms in its mesenteric vein. Thereafter, we repeated the same experiment with the A type cercariae, and confirmed each time that they developed into schistosome adults."——

The above story was abstracted and translated, in part, from their first two papers which appeared in a Japanese weekly journal. They also stated that,

"We were lucky, as beginners in this field, to have reached this conclusion. While we were waiting for the development of the larvae in the snail after exposure to the miracidia the days were very long and exhausing. We were always afraid of having the same experience as Leuckart once had, when he failed to obtain the full development of the larvae in the initial stage of his experiment with *Fasciola*, by using an inadequate snail host for the experiment. But, fortunately, the schistosome larva finally developed to the cercariae of the same type as we infected the mice."

At that time, the snail intermediate host of *Schistosoma haematobium* was still unknown. Before this, Looss made extensive surveys in the Nile Delta searching for intermediate hosts but failed. This presented the possibility that miricidia might infect man directly, and the larval development through sporocyst and redia would take place in the human liver. Miyairi stated that he was much concerned about this possibility, and at first he did not expect too much from his findings in the snail.

More comprehensive reports on the results of their studies were published by Miyairi (1914). He described the morphology of the snail intermediate host in detail, and classified it as belonging to the family Hydrobiidae. In Japan, the snail is now commonly called *miyairi-gai* (Miyairi's snail). The snail was named later by Robson (1915) as *Katayama nosophora*, under the following circumstances.

In February, 1914, a mission composed of Leiper from the London School of Tropical Medicine, and Atkinson, a British Navy Surgeon, was sent to the Far East to study the mode of spread of bilharziasis and to obtain if possible definite experimental evidence on this subject. They established headquarters at Shanghai, and stayed until the War broke out in August. Although they could not find the intermediate host while staying in China, this was achieved during the two visits to Katayama. Guided by Professor Fujinami, they collected numerous samples of the infected snail intermediate host, which had just been discovered by Miyairi and Suzuki. In their report (Leiper

and Atkinson, 1915), it was stated that, "The little village of Katayama is easily reached by ricksha run of about three quarters of an
hour from Fukuyama Station on the main line from Shimonoseki to
Tokyo. In a short space of time a large supply of this mollusc was
collected by the ricksha boy." On return to Shanghai, they teased
the snails in fresh water, allowed the "miracidia" (correctly, cercaria)
to become free and swim about, and then immersed mice obtained in
Shanghai. At this point, they had to go back home in view of the
outbreak of the War. However, all the mice thus infected died on the
voyage. When they arrived at Aden, they decided to sacrifice the few
molluscs that were still alive; the last remaining mouse was then
exposed to infection. This animal was safely transported to London,
where live male and female schistosomes *in copula* were recovered from
the portal vessels. The molluscs used in their experiments were submitted for identification to the British Museum, and Robson (1915),
in a note attached to Leiper and Atkinson's paper, described it as a
new genus and new species of the hydrobiid mollusc, *Katayama nosophora*. No reference was made to *Oncomelania hupensis* Gredler, 1881.
In this paper, Robson states, "That a freshwater mollusc occurring
in such great profusion should to all intents and purposes be undescribed is indeed extraordinary. Excluding the possibility of its having
been described in some inaccessible Japanese publication, we have to
bear in mind that it may have been recorded, through ignorance of
its anatomical characters, on conchological grounds as referable to
some other family."

[Like Robson states, it is indeed extraordinary, or rather unthink-
able, that a snail easily collectable in ample numbers by even a
ricksha boy, and playing such as important role, remained undescribed and neglected until then. Why could not Leiper and Atkinson
find it in China, where millions of Chinese farmers are now collecting
them as masses with a broom? Even stranger is, why Fujinami and
associates, or Miyagawa, or Tsuchiya, who had been working in the
fields for many years prior to Miyariri and Suzuki, did not recognize
this snail? I should have asked this question to Miyagawa, my professor in parasitology, who was the director of the Institute for many
years, before he died. However, while reviewing the classical literature, I discovered that a part of the answer to my question was given
already in an article by Miyagawa (1913 a), which was published
soon after the reports of the discovery of the intermediate host by
Miyairi and Suzuki appeared.]

Miyagawa (1913 a) stated that while carring on the experiments for infection of animals by exposure to the waters in the endemic area in Yamanashi in 1911, he had already believed that the intermediate host must be a kind of Mollusca, and collected various species. He crushed the snails and immersed rabbits whenever he found cercariae. From these experiments, he obtained two infected animals out of 11 rabbits exposed to cercariae obtained from "*kawanina*," (*Melania* or *Semisulcospira*), in July 1911. Since the infection rate was very low, he suspected that it might have been a contamination of the river water and did not publish the result. In 1912, he carried out an experimental infection of *Melania* collected from a non-endemic area, but the result was negative. However, he still suspected that *Melania* might be the intermediate host. By this time, he identified 8 species of cercariae in the snail, and exposed mice to each, but none of them developed to schistosoma. Then, on seeing Miyairi's article, he suddenly realized that he had confused *Melania* and *Oncomelania* (=*Blanfordia*) as a single species, and took it for granted that the latter was a young form of *Melania*. He states that the latter or the real intermediate host must have been contained in his sample, from which he previously obtained 2 positives out of 8. Miyagawa submitted the intermediate host (or his smaller form of *Melania*) for identification to Dr. Iwakawa, who examined it and stated that "this is a new and undescribed species of the genus *Blanfordia* A. Adams, and is closest to *Blanfordia japonica* Adams." (p. 1600, Iji Shimbun, 1913). However, neither of them named the species.

EPILOGUE

It was a long and painstaking course. It took nearly seventy years to solve the question raised by a country doctor, Yoshinao Fujii, who recognized the disease as different from all others he was taught from medical books, and who wanted to find measures for treatment and prevention. During the course of investigations, some workers were blessed with the discovery of either the parasite, the mode of infection and development, or the life cycle, but the tremendous efforts of many other workers ended in vain, or went astray.

With this story as a prologue, later workers in Japan devoted considerable time to discover effective measures for the prevention and treatment of the disease. As a result, the disease has been gradually controlled, and from about 1960 it became rather difficult to find clinical cases in all the endemic areas in Japan. In Katayama area, even the snail seems to have been eradicated some time ago. From 1970, the only places in Japan where the parasite and the snail are breeding prosperously are in some parasitological laboratories. As for progress in this field of research after 1915, excellent reviews were made by Okabe (1961, 1964), Komiya (1961, 1964) and Yokogawa (1970).

There is another important addendum referring to the above story. Leiper who visited China and Japan in 1914 and learnt about the snail intermediate host from the ricksha boy in Katayama, made an extensive study (1915–18) of African schistosomiasis in Egypt soon after his return from the Orient, and made outstanding contributions to knowledge in this field. He finally succeeded in determining the snail intermediate hosts of the two African schistosomes, which had remained unknown despite every effort of the past authorities. Futher more, Leiper proved the distinctness of *S. haematobium* and *S. mansoni* by susceptibility to the snail intermediate hosts, and his conclusions supported Sambon's idea of separating *S. mansoni* from *S. haematobium*.

REFERENCES

Baelz, E. (1883). Ueber einige neue Parasiten des Menschen. *Berl. Klin. Wochenschr.*, **20**, 234–238.

Catto, J. (1905). *Schistosoma cattoi*, a new blood fluke of man. *Brit. Med. J.*, **1905** (1), 1–13.

Faust, E. C. and Meleney, H. E. (1924). Studies on schistosomiasis japonica. *Amer. J. Hyg. Monograph Series*, No. 3, 1–339.

Fujinami, A. (1904). *Further discussion of the Katayama disease and its causative parasite. *Kyoto*, **1** (3), 13–25; *Tokyo Iji* (1380), 1842–5.

Fujinami, A. (1907). *Supplementary report on the description of Katayama disease. *Kyoto*, **4** (3) 220–231, (4), 233–265.

Fujinami, A. (1909). *On "Katayama-ki" written by Dr. Fujii sixty years ago. *Chugai*, (691), 55–56.

Fujinami, A. (1916 a). *Immunity to diseases due to macroparasite. *Kyoto*, **13** (3), 454–56.

Fujinami, A. (1916 b). *A history of researches on schistosomiasis japonica. *Nisshin*, **6** (1), 3–20.

Fujinami, A. (1916 c). *Pathological anatomy of schistosomasis japonica. *Nisshin*, **6** (1), 101–182.

Fujinami, A. (1916 d). *A catalogue of literatures on schistosomiasis japonica. *Nisshin*, **6** (1), 255–267.

Fujinami, A. and Kon, Y. (1904). *Pathology of Katayama disease. *Kyoto*, **1** (1).

Fujinami, A. and Nakamura, H. (1907). *Description of the habitat of *Schistosoma japonicum* in the body of animals. *Kyoto*, **4** (4), 266–267.

Fujinami, A. and Nakamura, H. (1909 a). *A report to the Research Committee on Endemic Diseases, Fukayasu-gun, Hiroshima-ken. *Chugai*, (707), 1153–63.

Fujinami, A. and Nakamura, H. (1909 b). *The route of infection and the development of the parasite of Katayama disease (schistosomiasis japonica) and its infection in animal. *Kyoto*, **6** (4), 224–252.

Fujinami, A. and Nakamura, H. (1909 c). *Serum reaction in calf experimentally infected with *S. japonicum*. *Kyoto*, **6** (4), 278–280.

Fujinami, A. and Nakamura, H. (1910). *Schistosomiasis japonica, its infection in horse, and the infective season *Kyoto*, **7** (2), 87–98.

Fujinami, A. and Nakamura, H. (1911). *On the prophylaxis of Katayama disease, and notes on its infection. *Chugai*, (753), 1009–27.

Fujinami, A. and Nakamura, H. (1913). *Observations on schistosomiasis japonica in various animals, with special reference to the horse. *Kyoto*, **10** (3), 262–270.

Fujinami, A. and Narabayashi, H. (1913). *Prevention of schistosomiasis japonica, especially the application of lime. *Chugai*, (794), 649–657.

Kanamori, T. (1898a). *Contribution to the etiology of tumors. *Tokyo Iggakai*, **12** (2)1 68–80.

Kanamori, T. (1898b). *On a new type of parasite egg. *Tokyo Igakkai*, **12** (3), 139–142.

Kasai, K. (1904). *Report of investigation of the so-called Katayama disease in Bingo, County. *Tokyo Igakkai*, **18** (3), 165–182, (4), 183–213.

Katsurada, F. (1904a). *On the endemic disease in Yamanashi Prefecture. *Okayama*, (173) 217–260; *Tokyo Iji* (1370), 1385–97, (1372), 1425–42.

Katsurada, F. (1904b) *Determination of the causative agent of a parasitic disease endemic in Yamanashi and several other prefectures. *Tokyo Iji*, (1371), 1442–6.

Katsurada, F. (1904c). *Schistosomiasis japonica in Saga Prefecture. *Okayama*, (175), 311–326; *Tokyo Iji*, (1380), 1823–34.

Katsurada, F. (1904d). *First supplementary report on schistosmiasis japonica. *Okayama*, (176), 361–369, *Tokyo Iji*, (1381), 1876–82.

Katsurada, F. (1904e). *On the geographical distribution of schistosomiasis japonica. *Okayama*, (178), 461–2.

Katsurada, F. (1904f). *A comment to Dr. Tsuchiya's article "On the so-called liver and spleen hypertrophic disease endemic in Yamanashi Prefecture." *Tokyo Iji*, (1377), 1687–90.

Katsurada, F. (1904g). *Schistosomum japonicum*, ein neuer menschlicher Parasit. *Annot. Zool. Japon.*, **5** (Pt. 3), 1–14.

Katsurada, F. *A contribution to the study of schistosomiasis japonica. Miura Moriharu Sensei Shushoku Nijushunen Shukuga Ronbunshu.

Katsurada, F. (1909). *Route of invasion of *S. japonicum* into animals, and the method of prevention. *Tokyo Iji*, (1928), 1686–9.

Katsurada, F. (1911). *Schistosomiasis japonica: Zoological aspects. *Byori*, **1**, 20–60.

Katsurada, F. (1914). Schistosomiasis japonica. *Centralbl. Bakt.* (I) Orig., **72** 363–79.

Katsurada, F. and Hasegawa, T. (1909). *Research on the development of *Schistosoma japonicum*. *Okayama*, (235), 433–443; (237), 1–7, German text.

Katsurada, F. and Hasegawa, T. (1910a). *Life history of *Schistosoma japonicum*. *Okayama*, (246), 470–474; *Tokyo Iji*, (1681), 1771–1774.

Katusrada, F. and Hasegawa, T. (1910b). Bemerkungen zur Lebensgeschichte des *Schistosomum japonicum* Katsurada. *Centralbl. f. Bakt.* (I) *Orig.*, **53**, 519–22.

Katsurada, F. and Hasegawa, T. (1913). *Supplementary remarks on *Schistosoma japonicm* with special reference to a new fact about the egg membrane. *Tokyo Igakkai*, **27** (2), 107–108.

Komiya, Y. (1961). *Prevention of schistosomiasis japonica. Nihon ni okeru Kiseichugaku no Kenkyu I, 99–129. Meguro Kiseichukan, Tokyo

Komiya, Y. (1964). Prevention of schistosomiasis japonica. Progress of Medical Parasitology in Japan I: 245–276, Meguro Kiseiechukan, Tokyo

Kurimoto, T. (1893). *Description of the eggs of a new parasite. *Tokyo Igakkai*, **7** (22), 1093–1098; **7** (23), 1159–67.

Kurimoto, T. (1904). *Hypertrophy of liver and spleen endemic in Yamanashi Prefecture. *Yokyo Iji*, (1334), 257–61.

Leiper, R. T. and Atkinson, R. N. (1915). Observations on the spread of Asiatic schistosomiasis. *Brit. Med. J.*, (1), 201–3.

Logan, O. T. (1906). Schistosomiasis japonica. *J. Trop. Med.*, **9**, 296–6.

Majima, E. (1888). *A curious case of liver cirrhosis caused by the eggs of a parasite. *Tokyo Igakkai*, **2**, 821–6; 898–901.

Matsushima, S. (1895). *A case of liver cirrhosis from the eggs of *Distoma pulmonare*. *Tokyo Igakkai*, **9** (13), 548–55.

Matsuura, U. (1909). *Report of investigation concerning the relation between schistosomiasis japonica and *kabure* (endemic dermatitis), and the route of penetration of the parasite into the human body. *Kyoto*, **6** (4), 253–265.

Matsuura, U. and Yamamoto, J. (1911). *Description of morphology of *Schistosoma japonicum* penetrating into the skin of animals. *Chugai*, (752), 937–939.

Matsuura, U. and Yamamoto, J. (1911b). *Description of *Schistosoma japonicum* in ditch water before attacking animals. *Chugai*, (755), 1153–5.

Mikami, S. (1900). *Hypertrophy of liver and spleen. *Yamanashi*, (3); (1901). *Yamanashi* (4).

Mikami, S. (1904). *Clinical symptoms of the endemic disease in Yamanashi Prefecture. *Tokyo Iji*, (1377), 1690–4.

Miura, K. (1904). *Demonstration of the liver and the spleen hypertrophic disease of Yamanashi Prefecture. *Tokyo Iji*, (1371), 1454.

Mirura, K. (1905). *Notes on Drs. Tsuchiya and Toyama's report of their investigation of the endemic desease of Yamanashi Prefecture. *Tokyo Igakkai*, **19** (10), 503–6.

Miyagawa, Y. (1912a). *Route of migration of *Schistosoma japonicum* from the skin to the portal vein, and morphology of the young worm at the time of penetrating the skin. *Tokyo Igakkai*, **26** (5), 3–4.

Miyagawa, Y. (1912b). * Relation between schistosomiasis and *kabure*. Method of fecal examination to discover the parasite eggs, and contribution to the knowledge of infection by this desease. *Tokyo Igakkai*, **26** (7), 5–6.

Miyagawa, Y. (1912c). Ueber den Wanderngsweg des *Schistosomum japonicum* von der haut bis zum Pfortadersystem, und ueber die Koerperkonstitution der juengsten Wuermer zur Zeit der Hautinvasion. *Centralbl. f. Bakt.* (I) *Orig.*, **66**, 406–416.

Miyagawa, Y. (1913a). *Concerning the cercaria of *Schistosoma japonicum* and the young worm at the time of its penetration into the body of the host. Contribution to the knowledge of the prophylaxis of the disease. *Iji Shinbun*, (890), 1512–31; (891): 1597–1608.

Miyagawa, Y. (1913b). Ueber den Wanderngsweg des *Schistosomum japonicum* durch Vermittelung des Lymphgefaesssystems des Wirtes. II. Mitteilung. *Centralbl. f. Bakt.* (I). *Orig.*, **68**, 204–6.

Miyagawa, Y. (1913c). Beziehungen zwischen Schistosomiasis japonica und der Dermatitis. *Centralbl. f. Bakt.* (I) *Orig.*, **69**, 132–42.

Miyagawa, Y. (1912). *Schistosomiasis japonica: Etiological aspects. *Nisshin Igaku*, **6** (11), 21–100.

Miyagawa, Y. and Taketomo, S. (1921). The mode of infection of *Schistosomum japonicum* and the principal route of its journey from the skin to the portal vein in the host. *J. Pathol. & Bakt.*, **34**, 168–74.

Miyairi, K. (1913a). *The intermediate host of *Schistosoma japonicum* and the prophylaxis of schistosomiasis japonica. *Tokyo Iji*, (1839), 2121–8.

Miyairi, K. (1913b) *Report of investigation on schistosomiasis japonica. *Tokyo Iji* (1850), 2747–52.

Miyairi, K. (1914a). *Description of cercaria of *Schistosoma japonicum*. *Iji Shinbun*, (895), 179–85; *Schistosoma japonicum* outside of body of mammals. *Nisshin*, **3** (9): 1315–51.

Miyairi, K. and Suzuki, M. (1912). *Contribution to the development of *Schistosoma japonicum*. *Tokyo Iji*, (1836), 1961–5.

Miyairi, K. and Suzuki, M. (1914). Der Zwischenwirt des *Schistosomum japonicum* Katurada. *Kyushu Teikoku Daigaku Igakubu Kiyo*, **1**, 187–97.

Mukoyama, G. (1902). *On the etiology of hypertrophy of liver and spleen in Yamanashi Prefecture. *Tokyo Iji*, (1252), 587.

Murakami, S. (1902). *Concerning the so-called new parasitic eggs of Drs. Kurimoto and Kanamori, and the endemic desease of Yamanashi Prefecture. *Tokyo Iji*, (1252), 577–8.

Nakahama, T. (1883). *Distoma hepaticum and Distoma pulmonale. *Chugai*, (72), 14–8.

Nakahama, T. (1884). *Morbus malarioides. *Chugai*, (111), 1–6.

Nakamura, H. (1910–1) *Pathology of schistosomiasis japonica. *Kyoto*, 7 (4), 239–82; 8 (1) 1–41.

Nakamura, H. (1911b): Schistosomiasis japonica: Pathological aspect. *Byori*, **1**, 1–10.

Narabayashi, H. (1913). *Morphology of *Schistosoma japonicum* at the early stage of skin invasion in animals and on its route of infection. *Byori* **3**, 363–76.

Narabayashi, H. (1914). *On the route of migration of *Schistosoma japonicum* in the body of animals. *Chugai*, (828), 1225–9.

Narabayashi, H. (1915). *Prophylaxis of schistosomiasis japonica, with special reference to the control of the intermediate host by the use of lime. *Chugai*, (855), 1381–1416.

Narabayashi, H. (1916). *Contribution to the study of schistosomiasis japonica. *Kyoto*, **13**, 231–78; 279–340.

Niizuma, Y. (1902–3). Study of the endemic disease of Yamanashi Prefecture, the hypertrophy of liver and spleen. *Chugai*, (536), 973–6; (561):

Oka, B. (1886). *A study on diagnosis and prophylaxis of an endemic disease. *Chugai*, (161), 1–11; (162), 12–21.

Okabe, K. (1961). *Biology and epidemiology of *Schistosoma japonicum* and schistosomiasis. Nihon ni okeru Kiseichugaku no Kenkyu I, 55–80.

Okabe, K. (1964): Biology and epidemiology of *Schistosoma japonicum* and schistosomiasis. Progress of Medical Parasitology in Japan. I, 185–220, Meguro Kiseichukan, Tokyo

Robson, G. c. (1915). Note on *Katayama nosophora*. *Brit. Med. J.*, (1), 203.

Stoll, N. R. (1947), This wormy world. *J. Parasit.*, **33**, 1–18.

Suzuki, T. (1895). *A case of pathological changes due to the eggs of distoma pulmonale. *Tokyo Iji*, (916), 1867–77.

Takegami, K. (1914) *Discovery of Schistosoma japonicum in Taiwan. *Taiwan Igakkai Zasshi*, (137), 183–201.

Tsuchiya, I. (1904a). *On the endemic disease of Yamanashi Prefecture, the so-called liver and spleen hypertrophy disease. *Tokyo Iji*, (1375), 1603–8.

Tsuchiya, I. (1904b). *Studies on the parasite causing the endemic disease of Yamanashi Prefecture. Part 1. *Chugai*, (592), 1513–33.

Tsuchiya, I. (1906). *On pathological anatomy of the endemic disease of Yamanashi Prefecture, or schistosomiasis japonica, with recovery of the parasite. *Tokyo Igakkai*, **20** (20), 763–805.

Tsuchiya, I. (1908). Ueber eine neue parasitaere Krankheit (Schistosomiasis japonica). *Virchow Archiv Bd.*, **193**, 323–369.

Tsuchiya, I. (1911). *Schistosomiasis japonica; Clinical aspect. *Byori*, 1, 11–20.

Tsuchiya, I. (1913a). *Concerning Drs. Miyairi and Suzuki's discovery of the life cycle of *Schistosoma japonicum. Tokyo Iji*, (1840), 2177–81.

Tsuchiya, I. (1913b). *On the intermediate host of *Schistosoma japonicum. Tokyo Iji*, (1850), 2733–7.

Tsuchiya, I. (1913c). *Studies on schistosomiasis japonica. *Tokyo Igakkai*, **27** (10), 725–86.

Tsuchiya, I. (1916). *Clinical aspects of schistosomiasis japonica. *Nisshin*, **6** (1) 183–254.

Tsuchiya, I. and Toyama, K. (1905). *Investigations on the so-called liver and spleen hypertrophy disease endemic in Yamanashi Prefecture. *Tokyo Igakkai*, **19**, 89–127; 140–173; 190–209; 335–357.

Umeda, K. (1909). *On the relation to *kabure* and microorganisms in polluted waters in the endemic area of schistosomiasis japonica, etc. *Okayama*, (234): 403–6; (235): 458–61; (236): 508–11; (237): 591–603; (239): 728–36.

Woolley, P. J. (1906). The occurrence of *Schistosoma japonicum* vel *cattoi* in the Philippine Islands. *Phillip. J. Sci.*, **1**, 83–90.

Wright, H. W. (1950). Bilharziasis as a public heatlh problem in the Pacific. *Bull. Wld Hlth Org.*, **2**, 581–95.

Yamagiwa, K. (1889). *Contribution to the etiology of Jackson's epilepsy (The pathological changes of the cebebral cortex caused by distoma eggs.) *Tokyo Igakkai*, **3** (18), 1025–42.

Yamagiwa, K. (1890a). *Histological reaction against parasites. Second report. *Tokyo Igakkai*, **4** (22), 1314–20.

Yamagiwa, K. (1890b). Beitrag zur Aetiologie der Jackson'schen Epilepsie. *Virchow Arch.*, **119**, 447–60.

Yamagiwa, K. (1891). *A case of liver cirrhosis. *Tokyo Igakkai*, **5** (7), 413–20.

Yamagiwa, K. (1909). On my mistake concerning the egg of *Schistosoma japonicum. Tokyo Iji*, (1636), 2062.

Yokogawa, M. (1970). Schistosomiasis in Japan in "Recent Advances in Researches on Filariasis and Schistosomiasis in Japan, pp. 231–55, Univ. Tokyo Press

List of abbreviations of Japanese periodicals:

Byori: Nippon Byori Gakkai Kaishi (Journal of Japanese Pathological Association)

Chugai: Chugai Iji Shimpo (International Medical News)

Iji Shimbun: Iji Shimbun (Medical News)

Kyoto: Kyoto Igakkai Zasshi (Journal of Kyoto Medical Association)

Nisshin: Nisshin Igaku (Medical Progress)

Okayama: Okayama Igakkai Zasshi (Journal of Okayama Medical Association)

Tokyo Igakkai: Tokyo Igakkai Zasshi (Jounal of Tokyo Medical Association)

Tokyo Iji: Tokyo Iji Shinshi (Tokyo Medical Weekly)

Yamanashi: Yamanashi-ken Igakkai Zasshi (Journal of Yamanashi Prefecture Medical Association)

Asterisks indicate papers in Japanese; English translations followed Faust & Meleney (1924) as closely as possible.

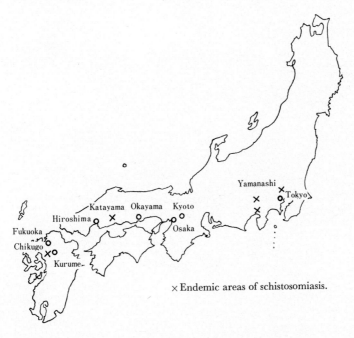

×Endemic areas of schistosomiasis.

Map of the Endemic Areas of Schistosomiasis in Japan